THE
LOW
FODMAP
RECIPE BOOK

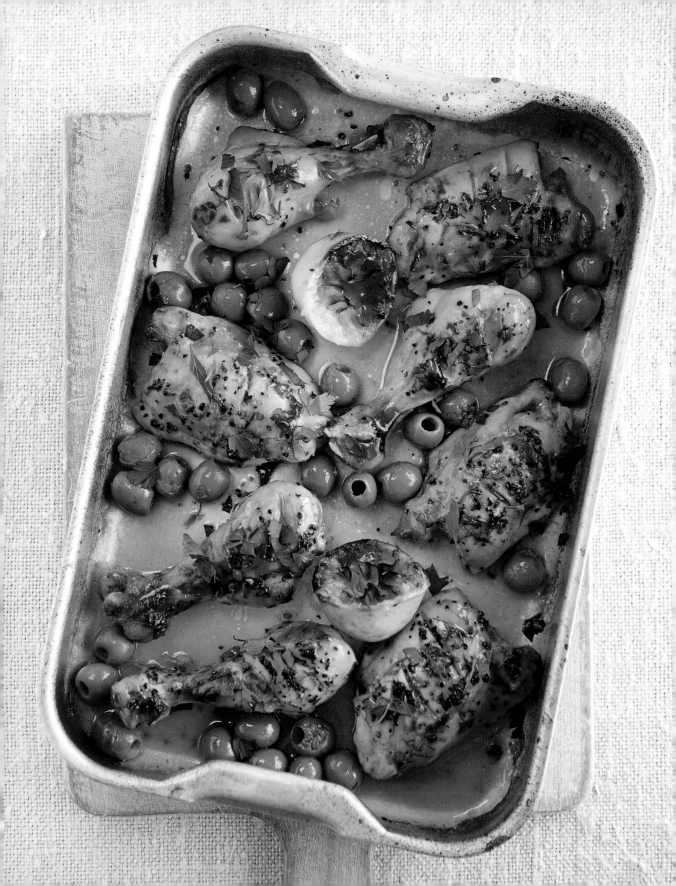

LUCY WHIGHAM

THE LOW FODMAP RECIPE BOOK

RELIEVE SYMPTOMS OF IBS, CROHN'S DISEASE & OTHER GUT DISORDERS IN 4–6 WEEKS

aster

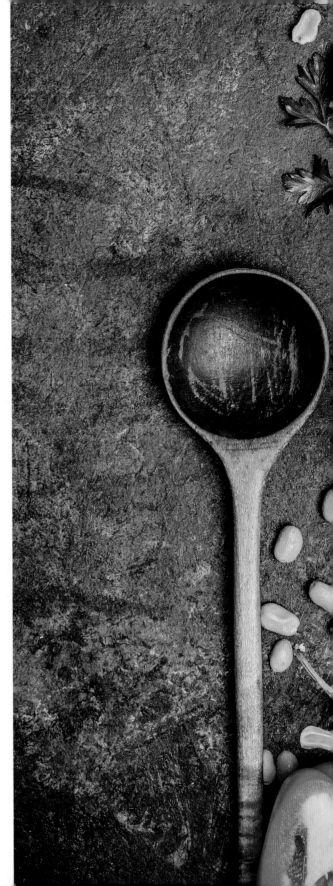

An Hachette UK Company
www.hachette.co.uk

First published in Great Britain in 2017 by Aster,
an imprint of Octopus Publishing Group Ltd
Carmelite House
50 Victoria Embankment
London EC4Y 0DZ
www.octopusbooks.co.uk

ISBN 978-1-91202-303-5

A CIP catalogue record for this book is available from the
British Library.

Printed and bound in China

10 9

Commissioning Editor: Leanne Bryan
Editor: Pollyanna Poulter
Senior Designer: Jaz Bahra
Designer: Geoff Fennell
Senior Production Controller: Allison Gonsalves

Disclaimer

All reasonable care has been taken in the preparation of this book
but the information it contains is not intended to take the place
treatment by a qualified medical practitioner. Before making any
changes in your health regime, always consult a doctor. You must
seek professional advice if you are in any doubt about any medical
condition. Any application of the ideas and information contained
in this book is at the reader's sole discretion and risk.

Cookery notes

Standard level spoon measurements are used in all recipes.
1 tablespoon = one 15 ml spoon
1 teaspoon = one 5 ml spoon

Both imperial and metric measurements have been given in all
recipes. Use one set of measurements only and not a mixture of both.

Ovens should be preheated to the specific temperature – if using
a fan-assisted oven, follow manufacturer's instructions for adjusting
the time and the temperature.

Eggs should be medium unless otherwise stated.

This book includes dishes made with nuts and nut derivatives.

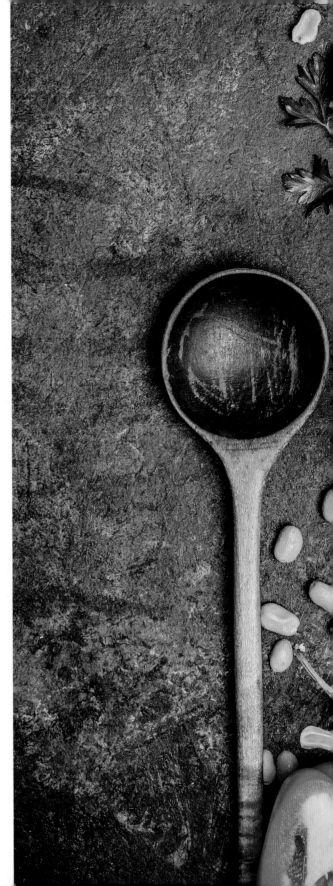

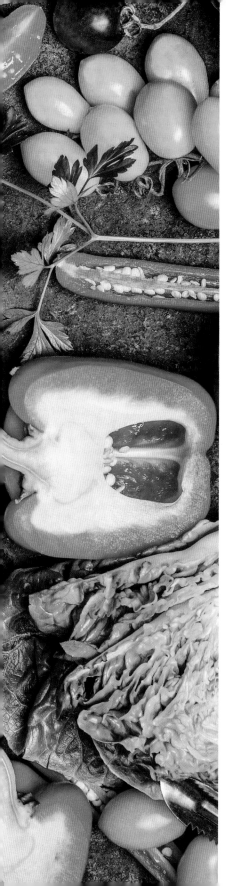

CONTENTS

INTRODUCTION

INTRODUCING THE LOW~FODMAP DIET

FODMAP is the current buzzword in the world of gut health and gastrointestinal distress. The low-FODMAP way can relieve even the most severe digestive discomfort. However, unlike most diets, this diet is not a fad. Rigorous clinical trials have proved the diet's effectiveness in treating symptoms of gut distress. Both the scientific community and the many people who have benefited from the diet are excited about its role in treating symptoms of IBS and other functional bowel disorders.

Around one in five people suffer from symptoms of Irritable Bowel Syndrome (IBS). Some experience the relatively mild yet disruptive symptoms of bloating and discomfort but, for others, symptoms are much more distressing, painful and embarrassing. A number of studies have shown that IBS significantly affects quality of life for sufferers, impacting on their enjoyment of social events and eating out, and increasing the number of sick days and visits to the doctor.

Medical treatments may help to ease the symptoms of IBS to some degree, but dietary manipulation is the cornerstone of treatment for the majority of sufferers. Traditional first-line treatment involving healthy eating patterns and regular meals with adequate fluid and fibre manipulation have limited success in resolving symptoms.

The low-FODMAP diet was developed by researchers at the Monash University in Melbourne, Australia. Researchers at King's College London, UK, pioneered further research on its use. Clinical trials have shown that, within four to six weeks, the low-FODMAP diet results in a significant improvement of symptoms in around 75 per cent of people who are diagnosed with IBS. These fantastic responses have led to the low-FODMAP diet becoming one of the mainstays of treatment for IBS across the globe, and it is considered the most effective way of treating the symptoms of IBS and other functional gut symptoms.

FODMAP
IS AN ACRONYM FOR
FERMENTABLE
OLIGOSACCHARIDES,
DISACCHARIDES,
MONOSACCHARIDES
AND POLYOLS.

WHAT DOES 'FODMAP' MEAN?

FODMAP is an acronym for 'fermentable oligosaccharides, disaccharides, monosaccharides and polyols'. These carbohydrates, present in a normal, healthy diet, are not fully digested and not absorbed in the small intestine and therefore go on to be fermented in the latter part of the bowel. This results in the production of gases and an influx of water, which, in susceptible individuals, causes pain, discomfort, constipation and/or diarrhoea and excessive wind. Lowering the intake of FODMAPs in the diet reduces the amount of gas produced and volume of water in the bowel, and can lead to substantial (many would say, miraculous) improvements in symptoms.

At first glance, the low-FODMAP diet may appear daunting, as the initial stage involves entirely cutting out or greatly limiting all five families of fermentable carbohydrates to begin with. These are:

FERMENTABLE...

OLIGOSACCHARIDES including fructans, found in wheat, rye, onions, garlic and various other grains and vegetables, and galacto-oligosaccharides, such as beans and pulses.

DISACCHARIDES which is lactose, found in animal milks, yogurts and some cheeses.

MONOSACCHARIDES which refers to fructose, found in various fruits, honey and agave nectar.

AND POLYOLS which are mannitol, sorbitol and xylitol and are found in certain fruits.

If you have IBS or another functional bowel disorder, are looking for a way to improve your symptoms and would like to try the low-FODMAP diet, it is important to consult your doctor before embarking on the diet and to work with a registered dietitian, who will guide you through the three stages of the diet (*see* page 14).

HOW THIS BOOK CAN HELP YOU

This book provides many delicious FODMAP-friendly recipes that enable you to follow the regime while ensuring a balanced, nutrient-rich diet. The recipes can be used during all stages of the diet.

There is no need to see the low-FODMAP diet as a mountain of boring restrictions. It can be something you can follow easily and with pleasure – and share with your family and friends – while your digestive symptoms diminish or even completely resolve.

Whether you need meals that are quick and easy to prepare, or you enjoy the art of cooking a dinner-party-worthy dish, this book will guide you step by step through the process of preparing tasty low-FODMAP meals…so you can have your cake and eat it (literally!).

WHAT ARE FUNCTIONAL BOWEL DISORDERS?

THE HEALTHY GUT

The gut or gastrointestinal tract is an amazing organ that carries out an array of important functions in the body, from digestion and absorption of food to defending the body from harmful bacteria and viruses. It runs from the mouth to the anus and each section has a different job to do. As food travels through the gut it is broken down into individual molecules using chewing and muscular contractions in the stomach and through the release of digestive enzymes from the mouth, stomach and small bowel. The individual molecules are absorbed across the gut wall into the blood stream and carried off to the liver for further processing and use in the body. Leftover waste continues down into the colon, where excess fluid and salts are reabsorbed, before the rest passes out as stool.

Food is pushed through the gut by muscular contractions that are controlled by a complex wiring of nerve messages called the enteric nervous system. This system communicates closely with the central nervous system (the brain and spinal cord) and there is a delicate balance between both, often referred to as the brain-gut axis.

There are tens of trillions of bacteria, of over a thousand species, that live in the gut. One-third of these species are common to most people, while two-thirds are specific to each individual (much like our individual fingerprints). Known as gut microbiota, these bacteria assist with healthy gut function and carry out many important functions, including digesting certain foods, producing vitamins such as Vitamin K, Folate and Vitamin B12, protecting the intestinal lining by fighting off invaders and forming a barrier effect, and playing an intricate role in the body's immune system.

Part of the role of gut micobiota is to break down undigested food that arrives in the colon, a process called fermentation. Fermentation produces useful by-products, such as short-chain fatty acids. However, it also produces gases. Some gases are absorbed by the blood and excreted through our lungs, while others remain in the gut and pass out of the body as 'wind', often without us even realizing.

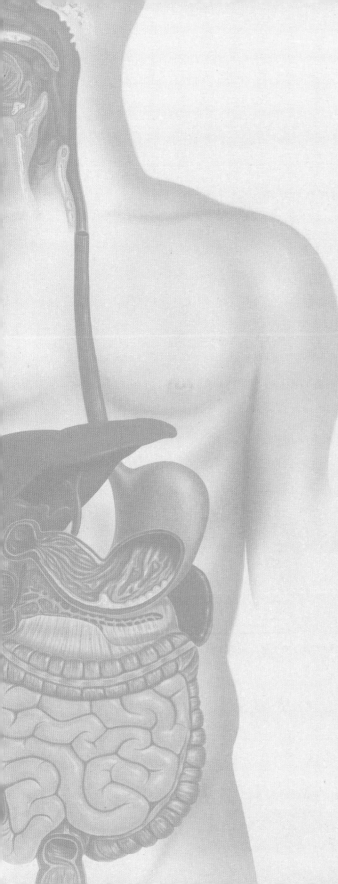

FUNCTIONAL BOWEL DISORDERS

In some people, despite the fact that there is no underlying structural abnormality in the gut, the functioning of the bowel causes abnormal symptoms such as pain, distension or bloating– so the problem is *functional*, not structural.

Irritable bowel syndrome (IBS) is the name given to a collection of functional bowel symptoms. It is characterized by an altered bowel habit (diarrhoea or constipation, or alternating between the two) accompanied by bloating, abdominal pain or excessive wind. Sufferers may also experience urgency to open their bowels, a need to strain when going to the toilet, feelings of incomplete evacuation after passing stool, fatigue, 'brain fog' and headaches.

The distressing effects of IBS can greatly impact on quality of life. For instance, the symptoms can make it hard for sufferers to even leave the house because of the frequency of necessary trips to the toilet. The pain can affect enjoyment of life and distract from work. Wind symptoms cause embarrassment.

Other disorders similar to IBS are functional bloating, functional constipation and functional pain. Along with IBS, these are collectively known as functional bowel disorders.

Symptoms are often worse after eating and around two-thirds of IBS sufferers perceive diet as being the main factor that influences their symptoms so they try modifying their diet. Many people embark on a frustrating cycle of restricting food groups without being sure which foods are causing their symptoms. It is common to approach social situations and meals out with trepidation, knowing that, in the majority of the instances, eating out will cause a flare up in symptoms, the causes of which remain a mystery. It is then easy to make the mistake of cutting out the food you think caused the problem when, actually, the cause was something else entirely.

POTENTIAL CAUSES OF FUNCTIONAL BOWEL DISORDERS

These are best described as a jigsaw of factors that interplay to cause a symptom profile for each individual. Not all of these factors will play a role in everyone's gut symptoms but it is likely that a number of them will be contributing to your symptoms. Let's look at these pieces of the jigsaw in more detail.

VISCERAL HYPERSENSITIVITY Visceral hypersensitivity, like many areas of functional bowel disorder, is not yet fully understood, but is thought to be affected by a number of factors including genetics, emotional stress and physical stress (such as a gut infection or gastro-intestinal surgery). As described on page 8, the gut is lined with millions of nerve endings that pick up messages from the gut and send them back to the brain. We know people with IBS have super-sensitive nerve endings, which means that the messages sent back to the brain are distorted or hyper- exaggerated, and are often interpreted by the brain as pain. The brain, in turn, 'speaks' back to the gut; how the super-sensitive enteric nervous system interprets these messages may result in spasms or changes in motility (the speed of transit and food through the gut).

GUT BACTERIA/MICROFLORA There is increasing evidence that changes or imbalances in our gut bacteria are linked to IBS and other functional gut disorders. We know that people commonly develop gastrointestinal symptoms after a gut infection such as gastroenteritis or food poisoning, often referred to as post-infectious IBS. At least part of this is thought to be due to changes in the balance of bacteria that live in the gut. People also sometimes experience a flare up of IBS symptoms after a prolonged or repeated course of antibiotics – again this is likely to be down to changes in gut bacteria.

GENETICS Your genes are likely to play an important role in how your gut functions. IBS and digestive issues often run in families – research points to a particular genetic mutation present in IBS suffers. It is likely that specific genes predispose certain people to IBS, and then environmental factors interact with these genes to trigger symptoms.

ANXIETY, DEPRESSION AND STRESS Research shows there is a strong correlation between anxiety disorders or depression and IBS/gut function. The majority of life stresses are unavoidable, but how we react to stressful situations can be modified. Some people are more prone to anxiety. Interventions that you may want to discuss with your doctor include counselling and psychotherapy, cognitive behaviour therapy, hypnosis, biofeedback therapy (see opposite) and medications. Things you can try at home that may help relieve anxiety, reduce stress and enhance your mood are regular exercise, addressing the work-life balance, mindfulness techniques, yoga and meditation, and finding ways to relax, such as listening to music or taking time each day to get some fresh air.

PHYSICAL STRESS Some people find their gut becomes more sensitive following a physical stressor, such as gastrointestinal or pelvic surgery, gastrointestinal infection, or a period of untreated coeliac disease or inflammatory bowel disease (IBD) flare up.

DIET Diet can impact on IBS symptoms in many ways. As well as FODMAPs, other factors in the diet, such as intake of fibre, fat, resistant starches and processed foods, can affect digestive symptoms. Your dietitian can discuss how these may be impacting you as an individual.

DISTURBED GASTROINTESTINAL MOTILITY Studies suggest that people with IBS sometimes have altered gut motility. Those with diarrhoea may have a faster-than-average gut transit time and those with constipation often have slower-than-average transit. It is not yet clear exactly why this change from the norm occurs, but it is likely be a result of messages from the central and enteric nervous system.

CO-EXISTING CONDITIONS Conditions such as fibromyalgia, endometriosis and bladder problems can all closely interplay with functional bowel symptoms. Getting the right treatment or medication for other health complaints may help your gut symptoms.

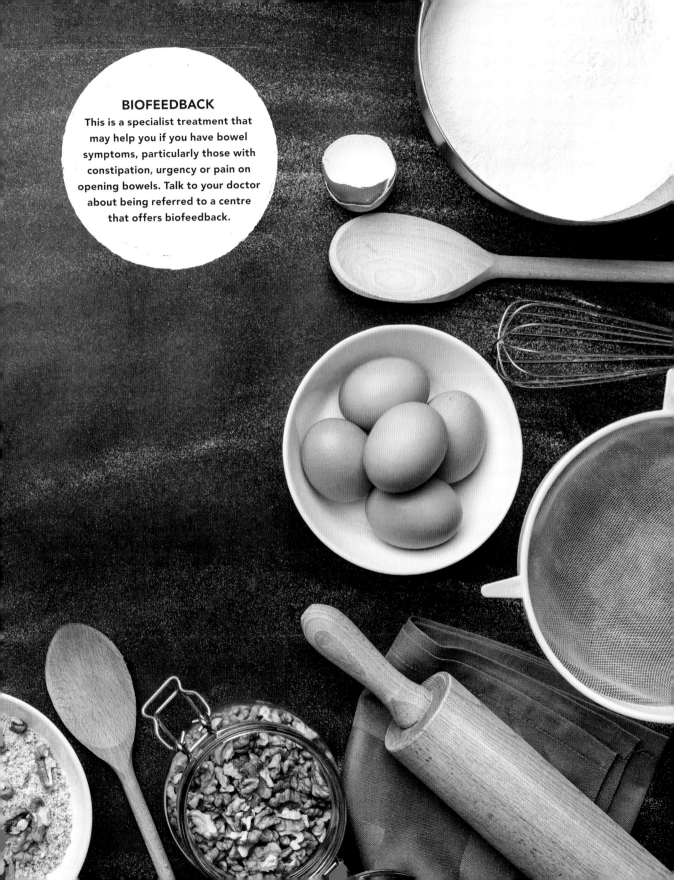

BIOFEEDBACK

This is a specialist treatment that may help you if you have bowel symptoms, particularly those with constipation, urgency or pain on opening bowels. Talk to your doctor about being referred to a centre that offers biofeedback.

HOW A LOW-FODMAP DIET CAN HELP

I have been seeing patients with symptoms of irritable bowel syndrome and digestive distress since 2006. People came to me with a variety of symptom profiles, from bloating and excessive, embarrassing wind that affected their confidence, to crippling pain and diarrhoea. We would spend time modifying their diets, trialling different exclusions, such as lactose and resistant starches, and adjusting their fibre intake. Often, symptoms improved with dietary changes but, frequently, they didn't improve enough for people to regain their quality of life.

The discovery of the low-FODMAP diet changed my life as a dietitian as well as the lives of thousands of IBS sufferers: finally, a dietary intervention that showed consistent results and improvements in global symptoms. Patients would come back after six to eight weeks on the diet and report that their symptoms had resolved and their lives had changed. Not only does my own clinical practice and that of hundreds of other dietitians reveal that this diet helps, but there are well-designed, robust clinical trials that have found that the symptoms of between 65 and 75 per cent of IBS sufferers significantly improve or are completely resolved on a low-FODMAP diet.

HOW DO FODMAPS CAUSE SYMPTOMS?

FODMAPs are a group of poorly absorbed fermentable carbohydrates that are present in our diets. Dietitian Sue Shepherd and Gastroenterologist Peter Gibson made a breakthrough in our knowledge of the link between these carbohydrates, diet and IBS symptoms in the 2000s. They termed the group FODMAPs.

FODMAPs aren't fully digested (broken down) in the gut and therefore can't be completely absorbed. So they remain in the gut, and their presence pulls in more water across the gut wall, which results in a higher volume of intestinal contents, which, in turn, can lead to diarrhoea and loose or frequent stools.

As these undigested carbohydrates travel towards and then through the colon, they meet with an increasing number of bacteria (our colonic microflora). These bacteria see the carbohydrate as a readily available food source and

ferment them rapidly. This fermentation process produces gas as a by-product; the volume of gas produced varies from person to person depending on the makeup of their microflora. In susceptible individuals – for example, those with IBS – this gas production can play a significant role in causing symptoms such as abdominal distension (in which the abdominal area becomes larger than normal), bloating (in which the abdominal area *feels* larger than normal), excessive flatulence, abdominal pain and spasms. It may also contribute to altered gut motility (the speed at which food passes through and is processed in the digestive tract), which can lead to constipation or diarrhoea, or often an alternating between the two.

Eliminating these fermentable carbohydrates from the diet or limiting their presence can reduce the volume of gas and liquid in the bowel, thereby improving the symptoms of gastrointestinal distress.

OTHER GUT DISORDERS

The low-FODMAP diet is a useful tool to consider using in the treatment in a variety of other digestive disorders as well as IBS.

INFLAMMATORY BOWEL DISEASE (IBD)

Inflammatory bowel diseases such as Crohn's and ulcerative colitis are autoimmune diseases characterized by intermittent inflammation of the gut wall. The low-FODMAP diet cannot treat the inflammation of the gut that occurs during a flare-up. However, many people with IBD also have a functional bowel disorder such as IBS, and their symptoms exist even when there is no inflammation of the gut wall. At times it is difficult to decipher which gut symptoms are due to a flare up of IBD, which require medical therapy and which symptoms are due to IBS. This is why, if you have IBD, it's essential that you work with your gastroenterologist and dietitian when deciding whether or not to embark on a low-FODMAP diet.

I have had huge success in using the low-FODMAP diet alongside medical therapy to treat those with IBD. However, it is important to note that people with IBD are more at risk of nutritional depletion than those without, so the involvement of a dietitian is key to success and safety.

COELIAC DISEASE Coeliac disease is an autoimmune disease that is characterized by the intolerance to gluten. This is a serious and lifelong condition that must be diagnosed by a doctor. Once diagnosed, the only treatment is a completely gluten-free diet, on which symptoms should improve.

Sometimes, despite sticking rigorously to a gluten-free diet, sufferers of coeliac disease are left with gastrointestinal symptoms, such as bloating and pain, even when their blood results show the disease is under control. These people are likely to have a degree of functional symptoms, possibly as a result of the gut being hypersensitive following a period of damage before the gluten-free diet was undertaken. In this situation the low-FODMAP diet may help address any residual gastrointestinal symptoms.

It's important to realize that while the low-FODMAP diet limits most sources of gluten, it is not a totally gluten-free diet, as it contains limited quantities of gluten-containing grains such as wheat, barley and rye, and allows gluten in the form of barley malt, oat products and small amounts of wheat as an ingredient in products such as soy sauce. The coeliac sufferer needs to ensure all low-FODMAP products and recipes are checked to avoid even trace amounts of gluten. Another important consideration in coeliac disease is calcium intake. Followers of the low-FODMAP diet have been shown to be at risk of not meeting their calcium requirements (see box, right), and as people with coeliac disease are at higher risk of low bone density, it is important to take extra care to meet your calcium requirements.

OTHER CAUSES OF DIGESTIVE SYMPTOMS

A low-FODMAP diet may help to treat symptoms of other causes of diarrhoea, such as bile acid malabsorption, microscopic colitis and lymphocytic colitis, by reducing the fermentable carbohydrates in the diet in conjunction with medical treatment offered by your doctor. The low-FODMAP diet may also improve abdominal pain and bloating after gastrointestinal surgery, but be sure to discuss this with your doctor and work with a dietitian.

BEFORE EMBARKING ON A LOW-FODMAP DIET

If you have gastrointestinal symptoms and would like to try the low-FODMAP diet, it is important to first consult your doctor and enlist the help of a dietitian to guide you through the stages of the diet (see page 14). FODMAP intolerances and gastrointestinal symptoms sometimes

CALCIUM

If you are avoiding lactose on the low-FODMAP diet you are at risk of having an inadequate intake of calcium. Some FODMAP-friendly calcium sources are:

- Naturally low-lactose dairy products, such cheese (see page 16 for more information)

- Lactose-free dairy products, such as lactose-free milk and yogurt

- Calcium-fortified alternative milk and yogurts, such as calcium-enriched almond milk

- Calcium-enriched orange juice (but stick to less than 100ml, 3½fl oz, per sitting)

- Firm tofu that has been made with calcium sulphate or calcium chloride (note that silken tofu is high FODMAP)

- Fish with small, edible bones, such as whitebait or tinned salmon

- Kale

feel like a moving target, as there are so many other factors that play a role in combination with diet. For this reason it is important to have guidance from an experienced dietitian.

Your doctor will ask you about the history of your symptoms and carry out screening, including checking for coeliac disease (you need to have been eating gluten for the coeliac screen to be accurate) and to identify any nutritional deficiencies and how to correct them. Your dietitian will consider your individual symptoms and test results and help you tailor the diet to suit you. He or she can help you get to know the lists of prohibited and limited foods, and also help you find ways in which you can adapt the diet to suit your lifestyle, likes and dislikes, and other dietary restrictions such as veganism, vegetarianism and coexisting allergies. As you progress through the stages of the diet, your dietitian will be able to troubleshoot for you if you find you are not responding to the diet, help you to interpret your response to the diet, and advise you on long-term management of the diet. Crucially, a dietitian can also liaise with your doctor on any medical management of your symptoms alongside dietary management.

FOLLOWING A LOW-FODMAP DIET

The aim of the low-FODMAP diet is to allow you to discover the specific triggers for your individual digestive symptoms. You will discover which FODMAP foods you need to avoid altogether, which you can consume in a limited amount and which you are able to eat freely. If you can understand how the things you eat affect you, you can establish a tailored, long-term modified FODMAP diet.

The knowledge you gain about which specific foods trigger your symptoms will give you choices by enabling you to weigh up how severe your symptoms will be and how long they will last with how much it suits you to eat that food in a given moment. For example, if you are at a wedding with little choice over the meal you are served and have a relaxing few days ahead, in which you can cope with any flare up of symptoms, you might decide to indulge. On the other hand, you might not want to risk a flare-up and will decide to stick more rigorously to avoiding all your triggers. The upshot is that the knowledge gives you more control over your diet and symptoms.

THERE ARE THREE STAGES TO THE LOW-FODMAP DIET:

1 THE ELIMINATION PHASE High-FODMAP foods are eliminated.

2 THE RE-CHALLENGE PHASE FODMAPs are reintroduced in a controlled way so you can identify the foods responsible for causing your symptoms.

3 THE MAINTENANCE PHASE You use the knowledge gained during the re-challenge phase to establish a low- or modified-FODMAP diet specific to you.

THE ELIMINATION PHASE

The elimination phase, sometimes called the restriction phase, lasts for four to six weeks. During this time, you discover whether or not your digestive symptoms improve when the quantity of FODMAPs in your system is decreased.

This phase entails avoiding all foods which are high in FODMAPs. Many people notice symptom resolution within a few days. For them, just four weeks is needed for this phase. Those who are a little slower to respond should persevere for six weeks to maximize their chance of seeing their symptoms improve.

People vary in how long they take to respond. Gut transit speed may play a role, and if you tend towards constipation it is likely it will take you a bit longer to see symptom response. Fermentable sugars can hang around in the colon for a few days. The after-effects of the fermentation process and activity of the gut bacteria can affect symptoms for longer than a few days. It has been suggested in one study that symptoms can occur for up to 30 days after ingestion of FODMAPs. For this reason you will get the best, most consistent response if you are as strict as possible regarding your intake of FODMAPs during the elimination phase. It is worth persevering. I have had clients who have not improved until week five, then have had the most miraculous change in their symptoms.

All five FODMAP groups must be avoided initially, because it is common to have a problematic response to more than one FODMAP family. Cutting them out one at a time often won't lead to significant symptom improvement because other FODMAPs that may be causing symptoms will still be present in the diet. (There are exceptions to this rule when it comes to fructose and lactose. See the information on page 16, and ask your dietitian for further advice.)

It is virtually impossible to cut out all FODMAPs present in the diet – that is why we call this the low-FODMAP diet, not the no-FODMAP diet. However, try your best to avoid all the foods that are high in FODMAPs. It is important to be as consistent as possible in the elimination phase.

HOW TO AVOID FODMAPS

The table opposite lists the foods that are restricted on a low-FODMAP diet. This is not an exhaustive list, as the understanding of the FODMAP content of foods is developing all the time. Your dietitian will provide you with the most up-to-date information on portion sizes and foods you can include or should avoid. Many foods contain more than one type of FODMAP, for instance cashew and pistachio nuts contain both fructans and galacto-oligosaccharides. For the re-introduction process you will need more information from your dietitian on how the groups overlap between foods.

What to AVOID and what to LIMIT

FOOD	AVOID	ALLOW IN SMALL AMOUNTS
VEGETABLES	• Asparagus • Beans (apart from green beans) • Cauliflower • Chicory root • Edamame peas • Garlic (including garlic puree, garlic salt, garlic powder, garlic flavouring – unless strained garlic oil) • Jerusalem artichoke • Leeks • Mushrooms • Onions (including onion salt, onion flavouring, onion powder) • Sugar snap peas • White part of spring onion	• Avocado • Beetroot • Broccoli • Brussels sprouts • Butternut squash • Cassava • Celery • Fennel bulb • Globe artichoke • Lentils • Mangetout • Okra • Peas • Savoy cabbage • Sweetcorn • Sweet potato
FRUITS	• Apples • Blackberries • Cherries • Figs • Goji berries • Mangoes • Pears • Stone fruits: peaches, nectarines, apricots, plums, prunes, dates • Watermelon	• Coconut • Grapefruit • Lychees • Pomegranate • Tamarind • Limit all other fruit to 1 portion per sitting
STARCHY FOODS	• Amaranth • Barley • Flours, breads, cakes, pasta made from the above grains • Rye • Spelt flakes • Spelt pasta • Wheat (trace amounts are allowed such as that in soy sauce)	
ADDED INGREDIENTS	• Agave nectar • FOS (fructo-oligosaccharide) • Fructose • Fructose-glucose syrup, fructose corn syrup, high-fructose corn syrup • Honey • Inulin • Oligofructose • Prebiotics • Sorbitol, xylitol and mannitol	
DRINKS	• Avoid all fruit juice from non-allowed fruit • Chamomile tea • Chicory • Coconut water • Dandelion tea • Dessert wine • Fennel tea • Oolang tea • Rum	• No more than 100ml (3½fl oz) fruit juice per sitting
NUTS	• Cashews • Pistachios	• All other nuts and seeds limit to a handful per sitting
DAIRY PRODUCTS	• *See* box on lactose intolerance on page 16	

FRUCTOSE INTOLERANCE Around 40 per cent of people don't absorb fructose, leading to digestive symptoms. It is difficult to know if you are in that 40 per cent. I usually recommend people avoid fructose in the elimination phase so that all bases are covered. Ask your dietitian for advice – you may have the option of being referred for a fructose breath test by your health professional to determine whether or not you are malabsorbing fructose. The best way to diagnose fructose intolerance is to avoid fructose for a period of four to six weeks, then reintroduce it and monitor symptoms.

LACTOSE INTOLERANCE Around 5 per cent of people of Northern European descent malabsorb lactose. The prevalence is higher in those of Southern European descent, and is even higher in those of Asian or African descent. If this malabsorbed lactose goes on to cause symptoms, this is called lactose intolerance (not everyone who malabsorbs lactose experiences symptoms). A lactose breath test can be helpful to determine lactose malabsorption, but the results need to be interpreted by someone with expertise in this area. As with fructose, the most accurate way to tell if you have a lactose intolerance is to cut out

LACTOSE
what to AVOID and what to CHOOSE

AVOID ON A LOW-LACTOSE DIET	SUITABLE CHOICES FOR A LOW-LACTOSE/LOW FODMAP DIET
• All animal milks including cows', goats' and sheeps' milks (unless it is specifically labelled as lactose-free)	• Plant milks such as almond, hemp, oat and rice • Small portions of coconut milk (less than 100ml, 3½fl oz) • Soya milk in limited quantities** • Specifically lactose-free milk such as lactofree™ milk (whole, semi-skimmed, skimmed)
• Yogurt	• Coconut-based yogurts (most on the market contain hidden FODMAPs but new brands are appearing all the time so keep your eye out and read the ingredients thoroughly). It is not clear what the maximum portion size of coconut yogurt is to ensure it is still low FODMAP so exercise caution and stick to small amounts, less than 3 tablespoons per sitting, and monitor tolerance. • Lactose-free yogurts (fruit or plain) • Soya yogurts ** • *It is important to check ingredients and avoid FODMAP fruits, added fructose, xylitol, inulin or FOS*
• Cottage cheese, cream cheese, halloumi, low-fat cheese, processed cheeses such as cheese strings and cheese slices, quark, ricotta	• Most other cheese including ripened cheeses like Brie and Camembert
• Custard • Ice cream	• Butter • Cream • Crème fraîche • Dark chocolate, small portions of milk chocolate • Soured cream • Soya custard and soya ice cream** • *You do not need to use special lactose-free butters, cream and hard cheese*

sources of lactose completely for at least four weeks, then reintroduce it using foods containing increasing amounts of lactose over a three-day period. This is often most successful when done alongside the restriction of other FODMAPs.

The recipes in this book are all suitable for a low-lactose diet (including the elimination phase of the low-FODMAP diet). However, if you know that you tolerate lactose well, you can use normal milk and yogurt instead of lactose-free or plant-based alternatives in the recipes, as long as you check the products you select for other FODMAP ingredients, such as FODMAP fruits or added fructose.

Most people with lactose intolerance can usually tolerate small amounts of lactose and that is why I recommend a low-lactose diet rather than a lactose-free diet. The table opposite gives guidance on what you need to limit to follow a low-lactose diet.

**Soya milk contains galacto-oligosaccharides and, although suitable for a low-lactose diet, should be restricted to 60ml (4 tablespoons) per serving on the low-FODMAP diet. It is not currently clear how much of these galacto-oligosaccharides are in soya yogurts and ice creams, but they are likely to be similar to soya milk and, for this reason, I would proceed with caution and limit to small portions only e.g. 2 tablespoons.

THOSE PESKY LABELS

You will need to carefully check the labels of any packaged foods you eat to ensure they don't contain foods listed in the avoid columns on pages 15 and 16. There are several low-FODMAP apps that can help with this (*see* Resources, page 244). I would recommend choosing one that is based on foods available where you live, such as the FoodMaestro low-FODMAP app produced with King's College London, that can be used in conjunction with your dietitian.

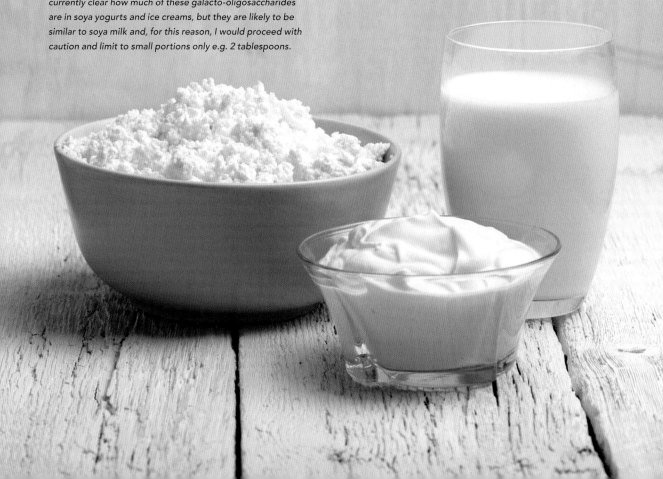

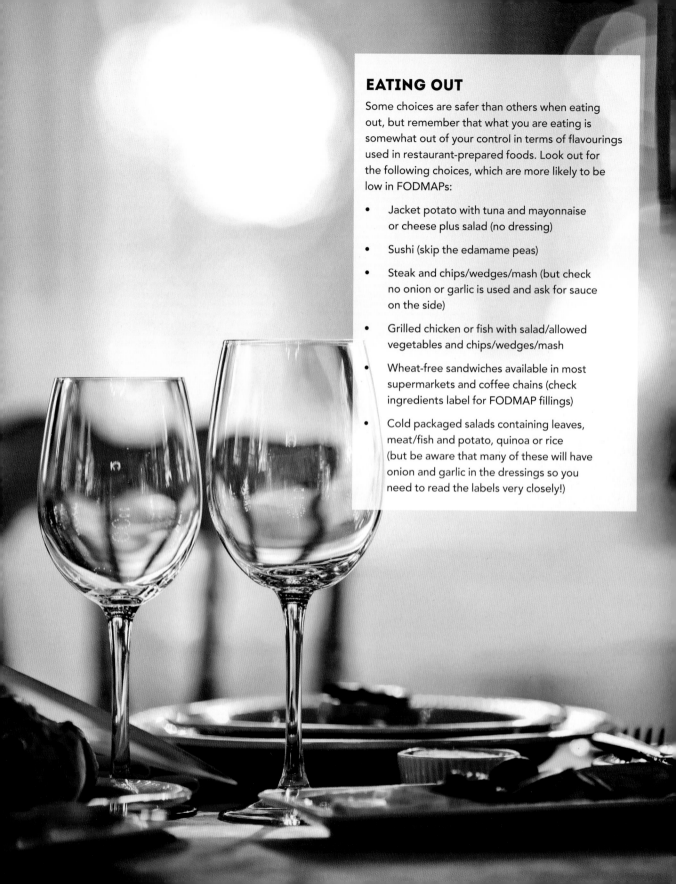

EATING OUT

Some choices are safer than others when eating out, but remember that what you are eating is somewhat out of your control in terms of flavourings used in restaurant-prepared foods. Look out for the following choices, which are more likely to be low in FODMAPs:

- Jacket potato with tuna and mayonnaise or cheese plus salad (no dressing)

- Sushi (skip the edamame peas)

- Steak and chips/wedges/mash (but check no onion or garlic is used and ask for sauce on the side)

- Grilled chicken or fish with salad/allowed vegetables and chips/wedges/mash

- Wheat-free sandwiches available in most supermarkets and coffee chains (check ingredients label for FODMAP fillings)

- Cold packaged salads containing leaves, meat/fish and potato, quinoa or rice (but be aware that many of these will have onion and garlic in the dressings so you need to read the labels very closely!)

WHY HAVEN'T I RESPONDED?

Some IBS sufferers do not get adequate relief from their IBS on the low-FODMAP diet. So why aren't you responding?

UNKNOWN FODMAPS SNEAKING INTO YOUR DIET Schedule a review with your dietitian to go through your diet to look for hidden suspects. If you don't have regular access to a dietitian you might find that keeping a food and symptom diary for one to two weeks, then looking back on it, can help identify if you have slipped up. Symptoms can last for between a few hours to a few weeks! So if you are slipping up weekly it could appear you are not responding to the low-FODMAP diet when, in fact, the failure to improve is due to not sticking to the diet. Remember to check ingredients on labels of anything pre-packaged. Especially beware of 'flavourings' that may contain onion or garlic powder and 'sweeteners' which may contain any of the polyols. Are you eating out a lot? To get the best out of the elimination phase, be discerning about how frequently and where you eat out during these few weeks, as hidden FODMAPs in restaurant food may be a contributor to not responding fully to the diet. Also, check your medication and supplements for hidden FODMAPs such as inulin, FOS and sorbitol.

EATING LARGE QUANTITIES OF THE 'FOODS TO BE EATEN IN MODERATION' There are a number of foods that are allowed on the low-FODMAP diet if eaten in moderation. But if you consume too much of these foods you give your body a high FODMAP load, so it's important to stick to the portion sizes suggested by your dietitian. You may find using the FoodMaestro FODMAP app (created by the low-FODMAP team at King's College London) in conjunction with information provided by your dietitian helpful in determining safe portions.

EATING TOO MUCH FRUIT IN ONE SITTING Even low-FODMAP fruit can cause digestive symptoms if more than 80g (2¾oz) is consumed during one sitting. The same is true for fruit juice. Limit fruit juices allowed on the diet to 100ml (3½fl oz) per sitting.

NON-DIETARY FACTORS ARE AFFECTING YOUR SYMPTOMS Two of the most common culprits for not getting adequate relief of your symptoms on the low-FODMAP diet are stress and anxiety. One scenario I often encounter is a client initially doing well in terms of symptom response on the diet, who then encounters a stressful week at work or family stress and sees their symptoms immediately multiply.

CONSTIPATION Sometimes people become constipated on the low-FODMAP diet and need to take extra steps to ensure good gut motility. Being constipated is likely to cause abdominal discomfort even if you are avoiding FODMAPs, so enlist your doctor's or dietitian's help to address this issue alongside doing the diet.

UNDERLYING PROBLEMS WITH GASTROINTESTINAL TRACT It is important to involve your doctor and dietitian from the beginning when starting on a low-FODMAP diet so they can rule out other disorders such as coeliac disease, inflammatory bowel disease, small intestinal bacteria overgrowth (SIBO), bile acid malabsorption, microscopic colitis and so on.

THE RE-CHALLENGE AND MAINTENANCE PHASES

Once you feel your symptoms are adequately improved after the elimination phase, your dietitian will take you through the re-challenge or reintroduction phase in a structured manner. In this phase you start re-challenging your gut with higher FODMAP foods by systematically introducing them, with the aim of identifying which FODMAP families cause your symptoms and how much of them you can consume before experiencing symptoms. This information is called your individual threshold level. If you need further information alongside your dietitian's advice, I recommend the book by Lee Martin RD on FODMAP re-challenge and reintroduction referenced in the resources section (*see* page 224).

Once you have established your individual threshold levels, your dietitian will help you to embark on the third phase of the FODMAP diet, the maintenance phase, which is often referred to as the modified FODMAP diet.

A FINAL WORD

The recipes in this book have been checked to ensure that the portion sizes are safe within the limitations of the ingredients, so it is important to follow the 'serves' info to prevent consuming too many FODMAPs.

BREAKFAST & BRUNCH

CONSUMING
1 TABLESPOON
OF LINSEEDS PER DAY
IS AN EFFECTIVE WAY OF
PREVENTING CONSTIPATION.
ENSURE YOU TAKE THEM WITH
A LARGE GLASS OF WATER,
TO HELP THE LINSEEDS
DO THEIR JOB.

PREPARATION TIME: 5 MINUTES
COOKING TIME: 25–30 MINUTES
SERVES: 2

600ml (20fl oz) lactose-free
or plant-based milk (limit
soya to 60ml/4 tablespoons per
portion), or standard milk if
you know you tolerate lactose

100g (3½oz) quinoa

½ teaspoon ground cinnamon

125g (4½oz) fresh raspberries

2 tablespoons mixed seeds
(such as sunflower seeds,
linseeds, pumpkin seeds and
hemp seeds)

1–2 tablespoons maple syrup,
to taste

QUINOA PORRIDGE
WITH RASPBERRIES

Bring the milk to a boil in a small saucepan. Add the quinoa and
return to the boil. Reduce the heat to low, cover the pan with a lid
and simmer for about 15 minutes, until three-quarters of the milk has
been absorbed.

Stir the cinnamon into the pan, re-cover and cook for 8–10 minutes or
until almost all the milk has been absorbed and the quinoa is tender.

Spoon the porridge into 2 bowls, top with the raspberries, sprinkle
over the seeds and drizzle with the maple syrup. Serve immediately.

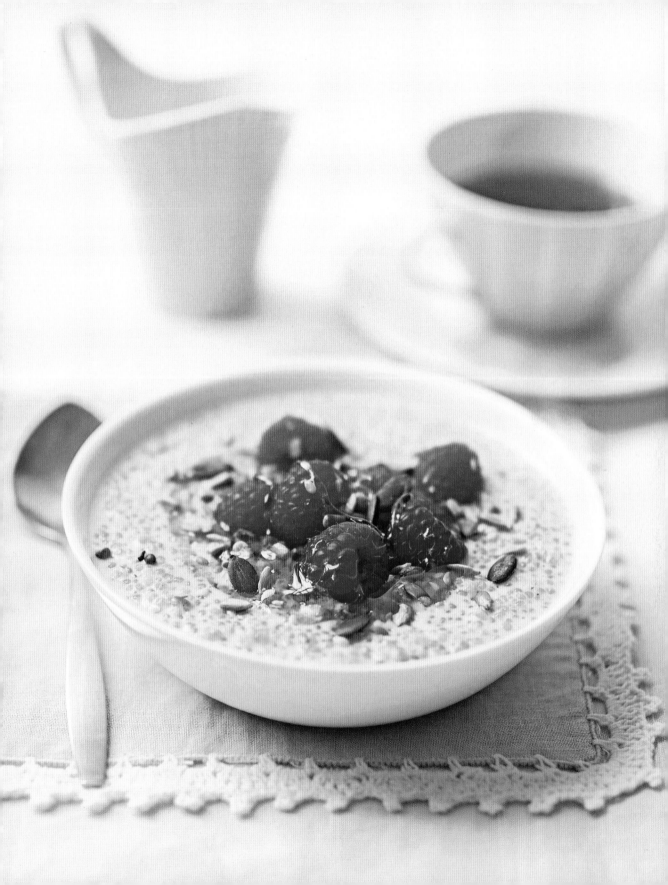

spray olive oil, for greasing

200g (7oz) porridge oats

80g (2¾oz) mixed low-FODMAP nuts (such as peanuts, walnuts and macadamia nuts), toasted and roughly chopped

1 tablespoon maple syrup, plus extra to serve

300ml (½ pint) lactose-free or plant-based milk (limit soya to 60ml/4 tablespoons per portion), or standard milk if you know you tolerate lactose, plus extra to serve

150g (5½oz) mixed low-FODMAP summer berries (such as raspberries and strawberries)

plain lactose-free or plant-based yogurt (limit soya yogurt to 60g/2¼oz per portion), or standard yogurt if you know you tolerate lactose

NOT ONLY ARE OATS HELPFUL FOR RELIEVING CONSTIPATION, THE SOLUBLE FIBRE THEY CONTAIN HELPS TO LOWER CHOLESTEROL AND STABILIZE BLOOD SUGARS, HELPING TO KEEP YOU FULL UNTIL LUNCHTIME.

SUMMER BERRY GRANOLA

PREPARATION TIME: 10 MINUTES, PLUS COOLING

COOKING TIME: 10 MINUTES

SERVES: 4

Preheat the oven to 180°C (350°F), Gas Mark 4. Spray a baking sheet lightly with spray oil.

Put the oats and nuts in a bowl and stir in the maple syrup. Spread out the mixture on the prepared baking sheet and bake for 5 minutes.

Remove the mixture from the oven and stir well. Return to the oven and bake for a further 3–4 minutes, until lightly toasted. Leave to cool.

Divide the granola between 4 serving bowls and pour over the milk. Add the berries and serve with yogurt and a drizzle of maple syrup.

BIRCHER MUESLI

PREPARATION TIME: 10 MINUTES
SERVES: 4

200g (7oz) porridge oats

100g (3½oz) mixed low-FODMAP nuts (such as peanuts, walnuts and macadamia nuts), toasted and roughly chopped

1 tablespoon maple syrup, plus extra to serve

600ml (20fl oz) lactose-free or plant-based milk (limit soya to 60ml/4 tablespoons per portion), or standard milk if you know you tolerate lactose, plus extra to serve

150g (5½oz) mixed low-FODMAP summer berries (such as raspberries and strawberries)

plain lactose-free or plant-based yogurt (limit soya yogurt to 60g/2¼oz per portion), or standard yogurt if you know you tolerate lactose, to serve (optional)

Put the oats and nuts into a bowl and stir in the maple syrup. Stir in the milk. Leave the mixture to soak for at least 2 hours or overnight in the refrigerator.

Divide the muesli between 4 bowls and serve topped with the mixed berries and yogurt, if using, with extra maple syrup for drizzling.

200g (7oz) porridge oats

600ml (20fl oz) lactose-free or plant-based milk (limit soya to 60ml/4 tablespoons per portion), or standard milk if you know you tolerate lactose

600ml (20fl oz) water

3 tablespoons freshly grated coconut

4 tablespoons plain lactose-free or plant-based yogurt (limit soya yogurt to 60g/2¼oz per portion), or standard yogurt if you know you tolerate lactose

200g (7oz) fresh berries (such as raspberries, blueberries and hulled strawberries)

4 tablespoons maple syrup (optional)

REMEMBER WHEN USING COCONUT TO LIMIT FRESH COCONUT TO 3 TABLESPOONS PER PORTION, AND DESICCATED COCONUT TO 1 TABLESPOON PER PORTION.

BERRY & COCONUT PORRIDGE

PREPARATION TIME: 5 MINUTES
COOKING TIME: 10 MINUTES
SERVES: 4

Put the oats into a saucepan with the milk and measured water. Bring to a boil, then simmer for 8 minutes, stirring often, until thick and creamy.

Pour the porridge into 4 warmed bowls. Divide the grated coconut and yogurt between the bowls and stir them into the porridge. Top with the berries and a drizzle of maple syrup, if using, and serve immediately.

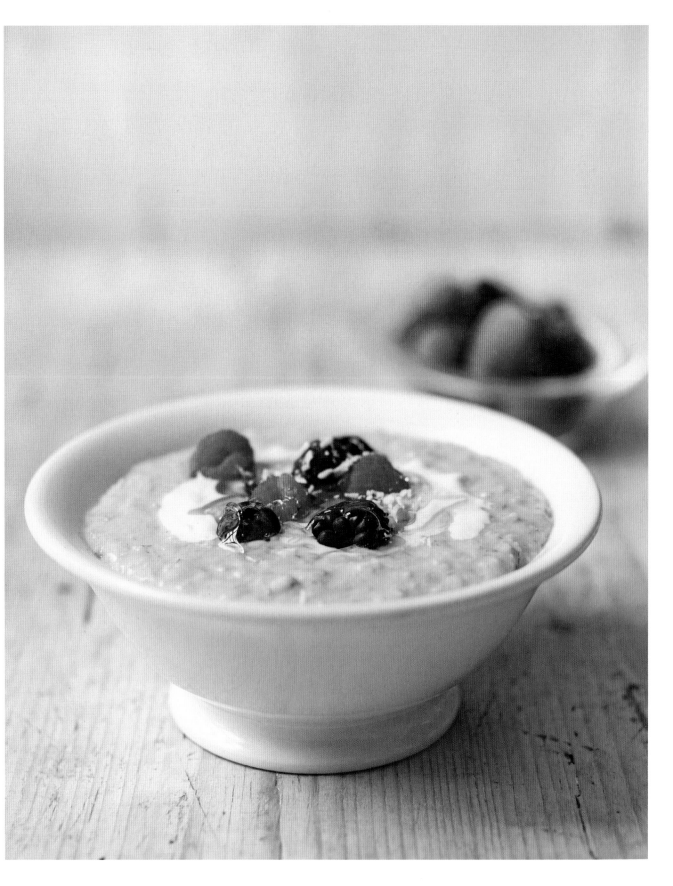

CUCUMBER, LEMON & MINT SMOOTHIE

PREPARATION TIME: 5 MINUTES
SERVES: 3

250g (9oz) cucumber, peeled
and roughly chopped

2 tablespoons lemon juice

3–4 mint leaves

2–3 ice cubes

strips of cucumber, to
decorate (optional)

Put the cucumber, lemon juice, mint leaves and ice cubes into a blender or the bowl of a food processor and process briefly.

Pour the smoothie into 3 tall glasses, decorate each with a strip of cucumber, if liked, and serve immediately.

1 ripe banana

300ml (½ pint) lactose-free or plant-based milk (limit soya to 60ml/4 tablespoons per portion), or standard milk if you know you tolerate lactose

1 tablespoon smooth peanut butter (free from high-fructose corn syrup)

PEANUT BUTTER IS A FANTASTIC SOURCE OF PROTEIN AND CALORIES, WHICH CAN BE ESPECIALLY HELPFUL IF YOU ARE STRUGGLING TO MAINTAIN YOUR WEIGHT ON THE LOW-FODMAP DIET.

BANANA & PEANUT BUTTER SMOOTHIE

PREPARATION TIME: 5 MINUTES, PLUS 2 HOURS FREEZING

SERVES: 1

Peel the banana and cut it into slices. Transfer the slices to a freezerproof container and freeze for at least 2 hours or overnight.

Put the frozen banana, milk and peanut butter into a a blender or the bowl of a food processor and process until smooth.

Pour the smoothie into a tall glass and serve immediately.

2 eggs, beaten

1 teaspoon vanilla extract

100ml (3½fl oz) lactose-free
or plant-based milk (limit
soya to 60ml/4 tablespoons per
portion), or standard milk if
you know you tolerate lactose

1 tablespoon caster sugar,
plus extra for sprinkling

½ teaspoon ground cinnamon

8 slices of gluten-free bread

25g (1oz) butter

fruit, to serve (optional)

> IF YOU WANT TO SERVE THESE WITH FRUIT, BE CAREFUL NOT TO OVERDOSE ON IT. AIM FOR A MAXIMUM OF 80G (2¾OZ) TOTAL FRUIT PER SERVING TO ENSURE EACH MEAL REMAINS LOW-FODMAP.

FRENCH TOASTS

PREPARATION TIME: 5 MINUTES
COOKING TIME: 5 MINUTES
SERVES: 4

Whisk together the eggs, vanilla extract, milk, sugar and cinnamon in a shallow dish. Place the slices of bread in the mixture, turning to coat both sides so that they absorb the liquid.

Heat the butter in a nonstick frying pan. Use a palette knife or a fish slice to remove the soaked bread from the dish and fry the slices over medium heat for 2 minutes on each side, until golden. Cut the toasts in half diagonally into triangles, sprinkle with a little caster sugar and serve immediately.

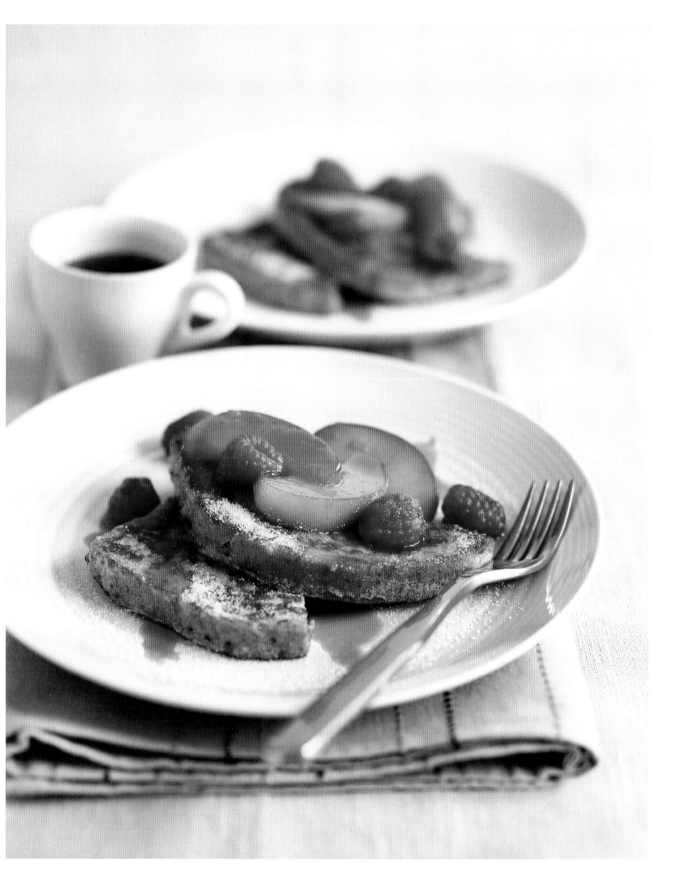

PREPARATION TIME: 15 MINUTES,
PLUS PROVING AND COOLING
COOKING TIME: ABOUT 40
MINUTES
MAKES: 1 LOAF

450g (1lb) buckwheat flour,
plus extra for dusting

3 tablespoons ground flaxseeds

1 teaspoon salt

1 teaspoon sugar

50g (1¾oz) psyllium husk
powder

3 tablespoons pumpkin seeds

575ml (1 pint) warm water

7g (½ oz) fast-action dried
yeast

2 tablespoons coconut or olive
oil, plus extra for brushing

GLUTEN-FREE BUCKWHEAT BREAD

In a large bowl, mix together the buckwheat flour, ground flaxseeds, salt, sugar, psyllium husk powder and 2 tablespoons of the pumpkin seeds. In a large jug, whisk the water with the yeast.

Pour the yeast mixture and oil into the flour mixture and mix well to make a sticky dough.

Tip out the dough on to a lightly floured surface and knead lightly for about 10 seconds, then return the dough to the bowl, cover the bowl with clingfilm and leave in a warm place for 30 minutes to rise.

Line a baking sheet with nonstick baking paper.

Shape the dough into a fat sausage, then brush it with oil and sprinkle over the remaining pumpkin seeds. Transfer the dough to the prepared baking sheet, cover the dough with a clean tea towel and leave to rise in a warm place for 30 minutes.

Preheat the oven to 220°C (425°F), Gas Mark 7.

Uncover the dough. Slash the top several times with a sharp knife and sprinkle over a little buckwheat flour. Bake for 35–40 minutes, until the loaf is golden brown and sounds hollow when tapped on the base. Leave to cool on a wire rack before slicing.

PREPARATION TIME: 25 MINUTES, PLUS 4 DAYS STARTER FERMENTATION, APPROXIMATELY 18 HOURS PROVING, AND COOLING

COOKING TIME: 40–45 MINUTES

MAKES: 1 LARGE LOAF

FOR THE STARTER

300g (10½oz) stoneground wholegrain spelt flour

350ml (12fl oz) cool or tepid water

FOR THE BREAD

400ml (14fl oz) warm water

2 teaspoons sugar

150g (5½oz) starter (*see left*)

500g (1lb 2oz) wholegrain spelt flour, plus extra for dusting

2 teaspoons salt

ALTHOUGH SPELT PASTA, SPELT FLAKES AND STANDARD SPELT BREADS ARE NOT PERMISSIBLE ON THE LOW-FODMAP DIET, 100 PER CENT SOURDOUGH SPELT BREAD IS. WHY NOT TRY MAKING YOUR OWN?

SPELT SOURDOUGH LOAF

To make the starter, put 100g (3½oz) of the flour into a plastic container. Add 150ml (¼ pint) of the measured water. Stir well to make a paste. Cover and leave for 48 hours.

After this time, small bubbles should have appeared on the surface. Stir in another 100g (3½oz) of the flour and 100ml (3½fl oz) water. Repeat this process 24 hours later. By day 4, your starter should be ready – it will be frothy, with large bubbles.

To make the bread, mix the warm water and sugar in a large bowl, then stir in the starter until well blended. Mix in the flour and salt to make a sticky, claggy dough. Cover the bowl loosely with clingfilm or a clean tea towel and leave to prove for 1 hour.

With lightly floured hands, stretch and fold the dough in the bowl, then cover loosely and leave to prove for 30 minutes. Repeat this process twice more, then cover loosely and leave to rise overnight or for about 6 hours, until the dough has doubled in volume.

Tip out the dough on to a floured surface and shape it into a round. Place it in a silicone bread maker or a preheated Dutch oven (if you cook it on a baking sheet, the loaf will spread out too much). Leave to prove for a further 30–40 minutes.

Preheat the oven to 220°C (425°F), Gas Mark 7.

Dust the top of the dough with a little flour and make 2 slashes in the top. Bake for 40–45 minutes, until the loaf is golden brown and sounds hollow when tapped on the base. If cooking it in a Dutch oven, remove the lid for the last 10 minutes of cooking. Leave to cool, then slice.

(You will have some starter left over after following this recipe, which you can use to make more bread if you keep it alive. To do so, continue to feed it by stirring in flour and water once a week, and store it in the refrigerator.)

125g (4½oz) gluten-free
self-raising flour

1 teaspoon gluten-free
baking powder

1 egg

150ml (¼ pint) lactose-free
or plant-based milk (limit
soya to 60ml/4 tablespoons per
portion), or standard milk if
you know you tolerate lactose

25g (1oz) unsalted butter,
margarine or coconut oil,
melted

100g (3½oz) blueberries

1 tablespoon olive oil

TO SERVE

plain or fruit lactose-free
or plant-based yogurt (limit
soya yogurt to 60g/2½oz per
portion), or standard yogurt
if you know you tolerate
lactose

maple syrup (optional)

BLUEBERRY PANCAKES
WITH YOGURT

PREPARATION TIME: 10 MINUTES
COOKING TIME: 20 MINUTES
SERVES: 4

Mix together the flour and baking powder in a large bowl.

Whisk together the egg and milk in a jug. Pour the wet mixture into the flour and whisk until the mixture is smooth.

Whisk in the melted butter, margarine or coconut oil, then gently stir in 75g (2¾oz) of the blueberries.

Heat the oil in a frying pan over medium heat. Spoon tablespoons of the mixture into the pan. Cook for 3–4 minutes until golden on the underside, then flip the pancakes over and cook for a further 2–3 minutes. Repeat with the remaining batter.

Serve with the remaining blueberries, a dollop of yogurt and a drizzle of maple syrup, if using.

YOU CAN REPLACE
THE GLUTEN-FREE FLOUR
WITH BUCKWHEAT
FLOUR, WHICH IS ALSO
A LOW-FODMAP FLOUR.

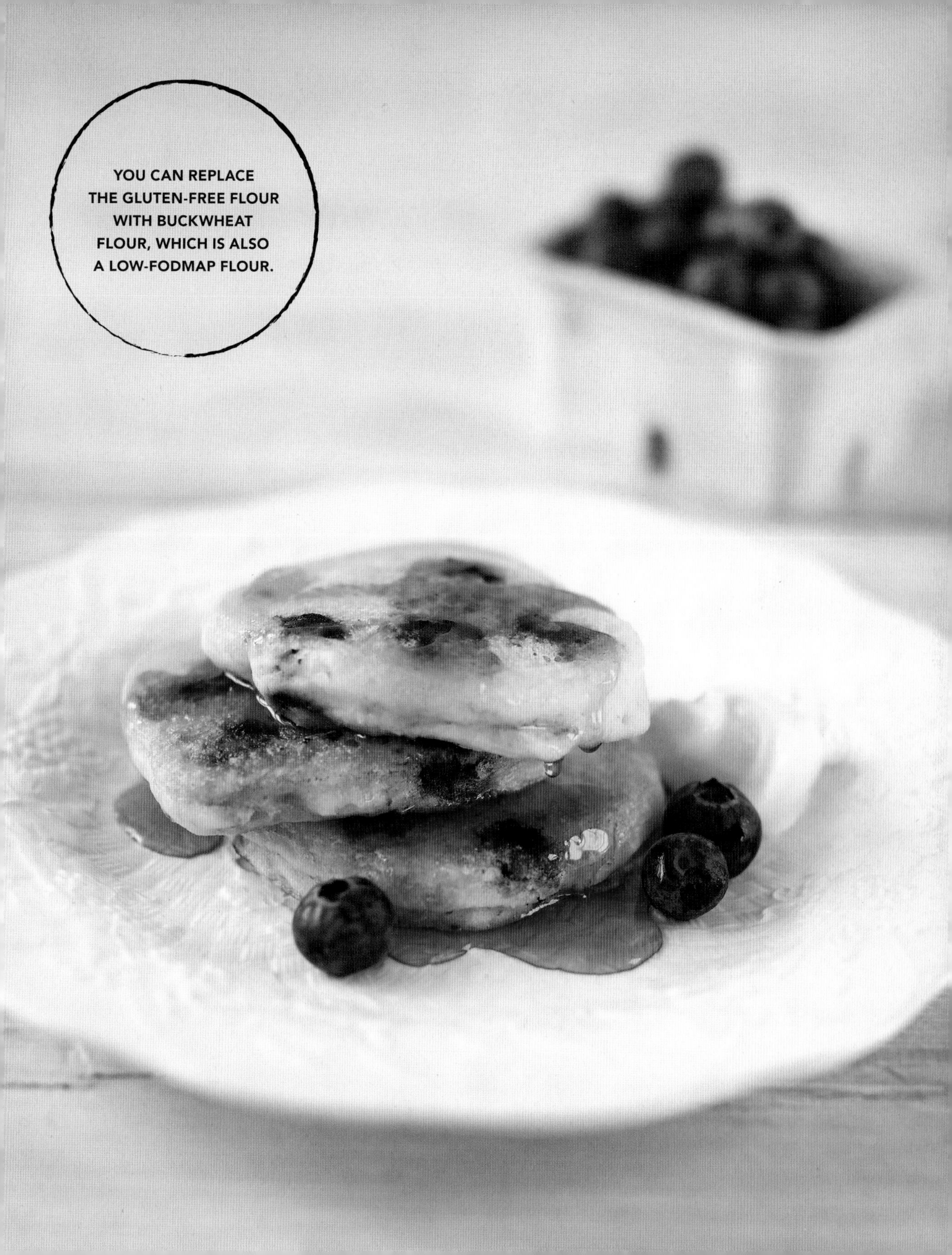

150g (5½oz) gluten-free
plain flour
....
150g (5½oz) gluten-free
self-raising flour
....
1 tablespoon baking powder
....
65g (2½oz) light
muscovado sugar
....
3 pieces of stem ginger
from a jar (about 50g/1¾oz),
finely chopped
100g (3½oz) frozen or
fresh blueberries
....
1 egg
....
250ml (9fl oz) lactose-free or
plant-based milk (limit soya
to 60ml/4 tablespoons per
portion), or standard milk if
you know you tolerate lactose
....
4 tablespoons vegetable oil

THESE MAKE
A GREAT ON-THE-GO
SNACK OR BREAKFAST AND
FREEZE WELL. JUST DEFROST
ONE OVERNIGHT AND SLING
IT IN YOUR BAG AS YOU
ARE RUNNING OUT OF
THE DOOR.

BLUEBERRY & GINGER MUFFINS

**PREPARATION TIME: 10 MINUTES,
PLUS COOLING
COOKING TIME: 20 MINUTES
SERVES: 12**

Preheat the oven to 200°C (400°F), Gas Mark 6. Line a 12-hole muffin tin with paper muffin cases.

Sift the flours and baking powder into a large bowl. Stir in the sugar, ginger and blueberries until they are evenly distributed.

Beat together the egg, milk and oil in a jug, then add the liquid to the flour mixture. Using a large metal spoon, gently stir the liquid into the flour until only just combined. The mixture should look craggy, with specks of flour still visible.

Divide the mixture between the muffin cases, piling it up in the centre of each case. Bake for 18–20 minutes, until well risen and golden. Transfer to a wire rack and leave to cool a little. Serve while still slightly warm.

GO EASY ON THESE AS THEY CONTAIN CRANBERRIES, THAT SHOULD BE LIMITED TO 13G (⅓OZ) PER SITTING AND NUTS AND SEEDS, WHICH SHOULD BE LIMITED TO A HANDFUL PER SITTING TO REMAIN LOW-FODMAP.

BREAKFAST CEREAL BARS

PREPARATION TIME: 10 MINUTES

COOKING TIME: 35 MINUTES

MAKES: 16

100g (3½oz) softened butter or coconut oil, plus extra for greasing

25g (1oz) soft light brown sugar

2 tablespoons golden syrup

125g (4oz) millet flakes

50g (1¾oz) quinoa

50g (1¾oz) dried cranberries

75g (2¾oz) blanched peanuts

25g (1oz) sunflower seeds

25g (1oz) sesame seeds

25g (1oz) linseeds

40g (1½oz) unsweetened desiccated coconut

Preheat the oven to 180°C (350°F), Gas Mark 4. Grease a 28 x 20cm (11 x 8 inch) shallow baking tin.

Beat together the butter or coconut oil, sugar and syrup in a large bowl until creamy. Add the remaining ingredients and beat well until combined.

Spoon the mixture into the prepared tin and level off the surface with the back of a spoon. Bake for 35 minutes, until deep golden. Remove the tin from the oven and leave the cereal block to cool in the tin.

Turn out the block on to a wooden board and carefully cut it into 16 fingers using a serrated knife. Store in an airtight container for up to 5 days.

4 courgettes, grated

4 tablespoons gluten-free
self-raising flour

40g (1$\frac{1}{2}$oz) Parmesan cheese,
grated

2 tablespoons olive oil

4 eggs

freshly ground black pepper

COURGETTE FRITTERS
WITH POACHED EGGS

PREPARATION TIME: 10 MINUTES
COOKING TIME: 20 MINUTES
SERVES: 4

Place the grated courgette, flour and grated Parmesan in a bowl and mix together well. Squeeze chunks of the mixture into walnut-sized balls and then gently flatten them into patties.

Heat the oil in a deep frying pan and, working in batches if necessary, fry the fritters for 2–3 minutes on each side, until golden.

Meanwhile, bring a large saucepan of water to a gentle simmer and stir with a large spoon to create a swirl. Carefully break 2 eggs into the water and cook for 3 minutes. Remove the eggs with a slotted spoon and keep warm. Repeat with the remaining eggs.

Serve the fritters topped with the poached eggs and sprinkled with black pepper.

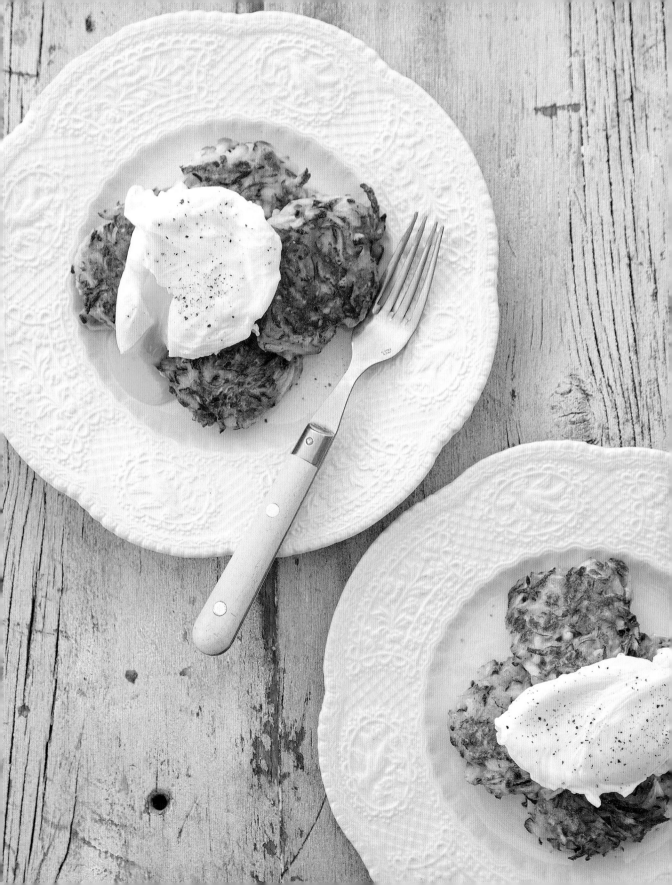

15g (½oz) butter or
1 tablespoon olive oil

450g (1lb) spinach leaves

pinch of grated nutmeg

4 large eggs

grated Cheddar cheese,
for sprinkling

salt and freshly ground
black pepper

FOR THE CHEESE SAUCE

20g (¾oz) butter

20g (¾oz) gluten-free
plain flour

¼ teaspoon English mustard

300ml (½ pint) lactose-free
or plant-based milk (limit
soya to 60ml/4 tablespoons per
portion), or standard milk if
you know you tolerate lactose

75g (2¾oz) mature Cheddar
cheese, grated

IT IS A COMMON MISCONCEPTION THAT ALL DAIRY PRODUCTS SHOULD BE AVOIDED ON A LOW-FODMAP DIET. CHEDDAR, AND MANY OTHER CHEESES, ARE LOW IN LACTOSE AND, THEREFORE, SUITABLE IN MODERATION.

EGGS FLORENTINE

PREPARATION TIME: 5 MINUTES
COOKING TIME: 20 MINUTES
SERVES: 4

Preheat the grill on the highest setting.

First make the cheese sauce. Melt the butter in a small saucepan over low heat, then stir in the flour and mustard. Cook, stirring continuously, for 1 minute.

Pour in the milk gradually, whisking to remove any lumps, then cook over low heat, stirring continuously, until the mixture begins to boil. Reduce the heat to bring the mixture to a simmer, then stir in two-thirds of the Cheddar.

Meanwhile, melt the butter or heat the oil in a saucepan, add the spinach and cook over medium heat for 3–4 minutes, until the spinach has wilted. Season with salt and pepper, then stir in the nutmeg. Transfer the mixture to an ovenproof dish or divide it between 4 individual ovenproof dishes.

Poach the eggs in a frying pan of simmering water for 4–5 minutes, then drain and place them on top of the spinach. Pour over the cheese sauce and sprinkle over the grated Cheddar. Place the dish or dishes under the hot grill and cook until golden and bubbling. Serve immediately.

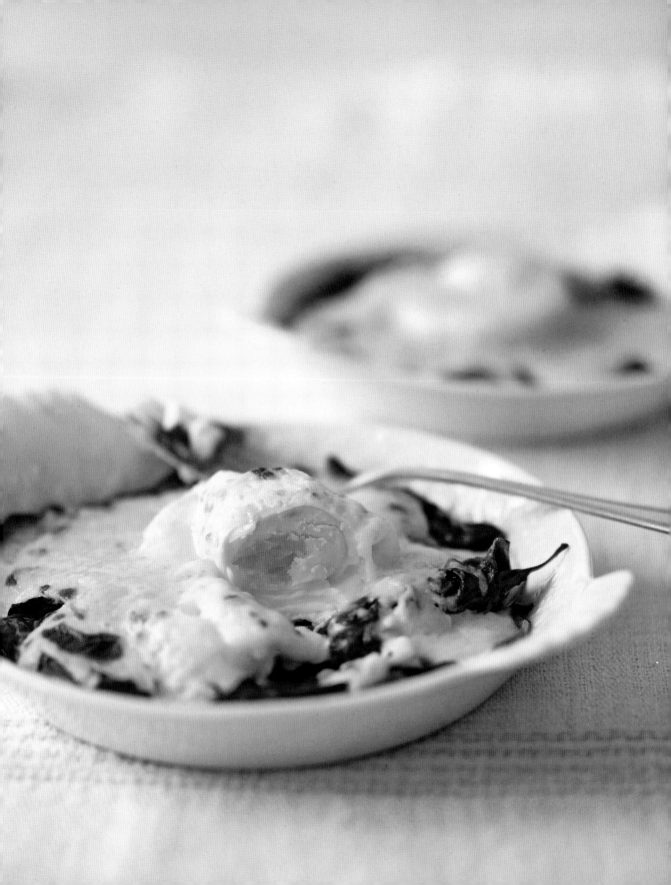

15g (½oz) butter
....
3 large eggs
....
1 tablespoon lactose-free or
plant-based milk (limit soya
to 60ml/4 tablespoons per
portion), or standard milk if
you know you tolerate lactose
....
1 tablespoon cream (optional)
....
25–40g (1–1½oz) smoked
salmon, cut into narrow strips
....
1 teaspoon finely snipped
chives
....
1–2 slices of toasted
gluten-free bread
....
salt and freshly ground
black pepper

SMOKED SALMON SCRAMBLED EGGS

PREPARATION TIME: 5 MINUTES
COOKING TIME: 3–4 MINUTES
SERVES: 1

Melt the butter in a saucepan over gentle heat until it is foaming.

Put the eggs into a bowl and beat well with a fork. Add the milk and season with salt and pepper.

Pour the egg mixture into the foaming butter and cook, stirring constantly with a wooden spoon, scraping the bottom of the pan and bringing the egg from the outside to the centre. The eggs are done when they form soft, creamy curds and are barely set.

Remove the pan from the heat and stir in the cream, if using, the salmon and the chives. Pile the mixture on to the hot toast on a warmed serving plate. Serve immediately.

275g (9¾oz) potatoes, peeled and chopped

30g (1oz) unsalted butter

60g (2¼oz) rice flour, plus extra for dusting

pinch of salt

1 teaspoon gluten-free baking powder

1 egg, beaten

2 tablespoons olive oil

TO SERVE

butter

300g (10½oz) smoked salmon

chopped chives

POTATO SCONES
WITH SMOKED SALMON

PREPARATION TIME: 10 MINUTES
COOKING TIME: 25 MINUTES
SERVES: 4

Cook the potatoes in a saucepan of boiling water for 10–12 minutes, until tender. Drain the potatoes and transfer to a bowl. Add the butter and mash together until the mixture is light and fluffy.

Sift in the flour, salt and baking powder, then add the egg and mix into a dough. Turn out the dough on to a lightly floured work surface and roll it out to a thickness of about 5mm (¼ inch). Cut the dough into 8 wedges and prick them all over with a fork.

Heat the oil in a large frying pan over medium heat. Add the wedges and cook for 4–5 minutes on each side, until golden. Transfer to serving plates.

To serve, spread each scone with a little butter, top with smoked salmon and sprinkle over some chopped chives.

2 tablespoons garlic-infused
olive oil

2 red peppers, deseeded
and diced

1 bunch of spring onions
(green parts only), sliced

¾ teaspoon dried oregano

400g (14oz) can chopped
tomatoes

4 eggs

20g (¾oz) feta cheese,
crumbled

4 toasted gluten-free pitta
breads, to serve

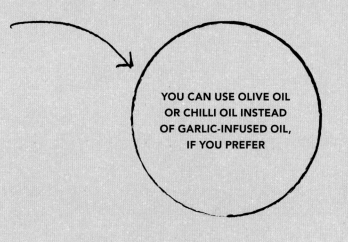

YOU CAN USE OLIVE OIL
OR CHILLI OIL INSTEAD
OF GARLIC-INFUSED OIL,
IF YOU PREFER

HUEVOS RANCHEROS

PREPARATION TIME: 5 MINUTES
COOKING TIME: 15 MINUTES
SERVES: 4

Preheat the grill on the highest setting.

Heat the oil in a frying pan over medium heat. Add the peppers and cook for 3–4 minutes, until softened. Add the spring onion and oregano and cook for 1 minute. Add the tomatoes and cook for a further 5 minutes. Pour the tomato mixture into a shallow ovenproof dish. Use the back of a spoon to make 4 dips, evenly spaced, in the mixture.

Crack the eggs into the dips in the tomato mixture, then sprinkle over the feta. Cook under the hot grill for 3–4 minutes or until the eggs are cooked to your liking. Serve with toasted pitta breads.

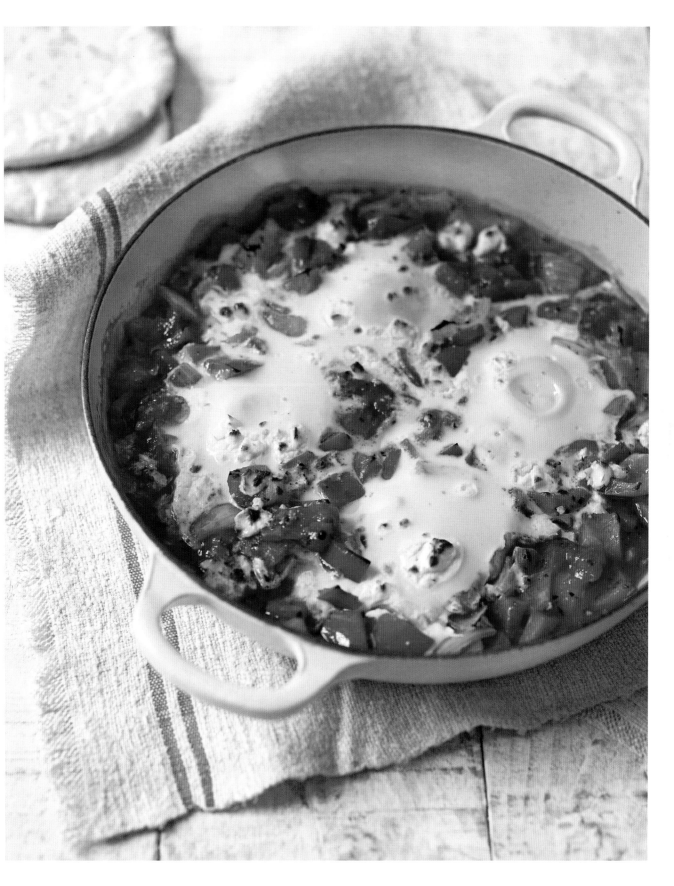

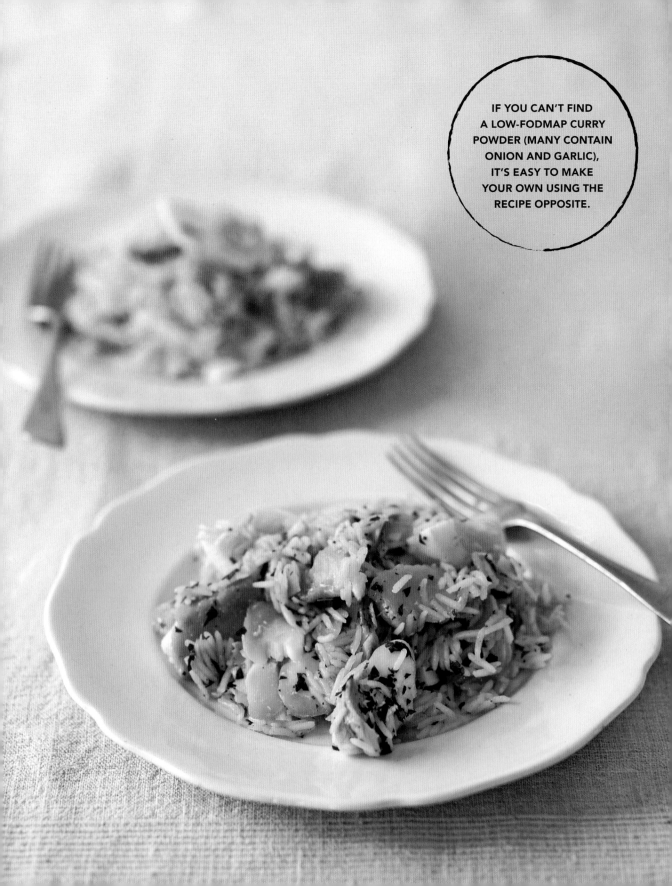

IF YOU CAN'T FIND
A LOW-FODMAP CURRY
POWDER (MANY CONTAIN
ONION AND GARLIC),
IT'S EASY TO MAKE
YOUR OWN USING THE
RECIPE OPPOSITE.

KEDGEREE

Place the haddock in a saucepan and cover with the measured water. Bring to a simmer, cover the pan with a lid and cook over medium heat for 8–10 minutes. Drain the fish, reserving the cooking liquid, and keep the fish warm.

Heat the oil in the same saucepan you used to cook the fish, then add the spring onion and cook for 1–2 minutes, until softened. Stir in the curry powder, then the rice.

Pour in 450ml (16fl oz) of the reserved cooking liquid and bring to a simmer, then cover the pan with a lid and cook for 15 minutes or until the rice is tender and the water has been absorbed.

Skin and flake the fish and carefully stir it into the rice with the quartered eggs.

Serve sprinkled with chopped parsley and a squeeze of lemon juice.

PREPARATION TIME: 10 MINUTES
COOKING TIME: 30 MINUTES
SERVES: 4

500g (1lb 2oz) smoked haddock

600ml (20fl oz) water

50ml (2fl oz) olive oil or rapeseed oil

1 bunch of spring onions (green parts only), sliced

¾ teaspoon mild Low-FODMAP Curry Powder (see below)

225g (8oz) basmati rice

4 eggs, hard-boiled, shelled and quartered

2 tablespoons chopped flat-leaf parsley

2 tablespoons lemon juice

LOW-FODMAP CURRY POWDER

Ensure that the curry powder you use is FODMAP friendly – many products contain onion and garlic, which should be avoided in a low-FODMAP diet. If you can't find a low-FODMAP curry powder, you might like to make your own using the following recipe.

Combine 2 tablespoons each of ground cardamom, ground coriander, ground cumin, turmeric and mustard powder with 1 teaspoon each of ground ginger and ground cinnamon, and ¼–2 teaspoons of cayenne pepper (depending on how hot you like your curries). Store in an airtight container.

LUNCHES

CHICKEN CLUB SANDWICH ⟶

Heat the oil in a nonstick frying pan. Add the chicken and bacon and fry over medium heat for 6–8 minutes, turning once or twice, until golden and cooked through.

Toast the bread on both sides, then spread 1 side of each piece with the mayonnaise. Divide the chicken and bacon across 4 slices of the toast, then top with the sliced cheese. Cover the cheese with 4 more slices of toast, then add the tomato slices and watercress. Complete the sandwich stacks with the final slices of toast.

Press the sandwiches together, then cut each stack into 4 small triangles. Secure with cocktail sticks, if needed, and serve immediately.

PREPARATION TIME: 15 MINUTES
COOKING TIME: 10 MINUTES
SERVES: 4

1 tablespoon sunflower oil
....
4 small boneless, skinless chicken breasts, thinly sliced
....
8 smoked back bacon rashers
....
12 slices of gluten-free bread
....
4 tablespoons mayonnaise (free from garlic and onion)
....
125g (4½oz) blue cheese, thinly sliced
....
4 vine tomatoes, thinly sliced
....
40g (1½oz) watercress

BLT SANDWICH

PREPARATION TIME: 5 MINUTES
COOKING TIME: 5 MINUTES
SERVES: 1

2 lean bacon rashers
....
2 slices of gluten-free brown bread
....
2 tablespoons mayonnaise (free from garlic and onion)
....
2 vine tomatoes, halved
....
about 4 little gem lettuce leaves
....
salt and freshly ground black pepper

Heat a small nonstick frying pan and cook the bacon over medium heat for about 5 minutes, turning once, until it is golden brown and crisp. Remove and drain on kitchen paper.

Toast the bread on both sides. Spread 1 side of each piece of toast with mayonnaise and arrange the bacon, tomatoes and lettuce on top. Season with salt and pepper and top with the remaining piece of toast. Cut the sandwich into quarters. Serve hot or cold.

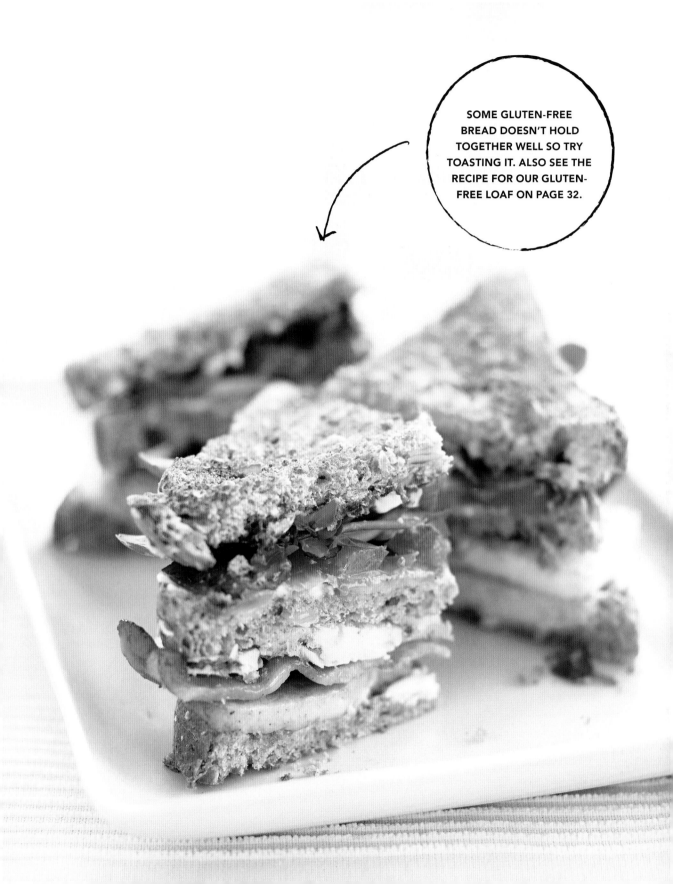

SOME GLUTEN-FREE BREAD DOESN'T HOLD TOGETHER WELL SO TRY TOASTING IT. ALSO SEE THE RECIPE FOR OUR GLUTEN-FREE LOAF ON PAGE 32.

500g (1lb 2oz) thick sirloin
steak, trimmed

1 tablespoon olive oil

4 gluten-free mini baguettes
or bread rolls, split open

4 sprigs of fresh coriander

4 sprigs of basil or Thai
basil

4 sprigs of mint

salt and freshly ground
black pepper

FOR THE DRESSING

2 tablespoons Thai fish sauce

2 tablespoons lime juice

2 tablespoons soft light
brown sugar

1 large red chilli, thinly
sliced

CHILLI THAI BEEF BAGUETTES

**PREPARATION TIME: 5 MINUTES,
PLUS RESTING
COOKING TIME: 4 MINUTES
SERVES: 4**

Heat a griddle pan until very hot.

Brush the steak with the oil and season liberally with salt and pepper. Add the steak to the hot griddle pan and cook over high heat for 2 minutes on each side, ensuring you sear the steak all over. Leave to rest for 5 minutes, then cut it into thin slices. The steak should be rare.

Meanwhile, make the dressing. Put the fish sauce, lime juice and sugar into a bowl and stir in the chilli until the sugar has dissolved.

Fill the split rolls with the herbs and the beef slices along with any juices. Carefully pour over the dressing and serve.

200g (7oz) rice noodles

1 bunch of spring onions (green parts only), thinly sliced

15mm (¾inch) piece of fresh root ginger, peeled and grated

1 red chilli, finely chopped

2 tablespoons chopped fresh coriander

1 tablespoon chopped mint

¼ cucumber, cut into fine matchsticks

2 x 175g (6oz) cans crabmeat, drained, or 300g (10½oz) fresh white crabmeat

1 tablespoon sesame oil

1 teaspoon Thai fish sauce

16 rice paper wrappers

THE WHITE BULBS OF SPRING ONIONS ARE HIGH IN FODMAPS SO BE SURE TO USE THE GREEN PARTS ONLY.

CRAB & NOODLE ASIAN WRAPS

PREPARATION TIME: 15 MINUTES, PLUS STANDING
COOKING TIME: 5 MINUTES
SERVES: 4

Cook the rice noodles according to the packet instructions. Drain the noodles, then refresh under cold running water.

Mix together the remaining ingredients, except the rice paper wrappers, in a large bowl. Add the noodles and toss to mix. Cover and set aside for 10 minutes to allow the flavours to develop, then transfer to a serving dish.

Serve the filling mixture in a bowl alongside the rice paper wrappers and a bowl of warm water. Allow 4 rice paper wrappers per person and allow diners to soak and then top each wrapper with some of the crab and noodle mixture, roll it up and enjoy.

PREPARATION TIME: 15 MINUTES,
    PLUS COOLING
COOKING TIME: ABOUT
    15 MINUTES
SERVES: 4

300g (10½oz) sushi rice
....
2 tablespoons rice wine
vinegar
....
1 tablespoon caster sugar
....
2 sheets of nori
....
1 teaspoon wasabi
....
2 long strips of cucumber,
cut to the length of the
nori sheet and about 1cm
(½ inch) thick
....
100g (3½oz) smoked salmon
....
2 tablespoons Japanese
pickled ginger
....
4 tablespoons light soy sauce

SALMON & CUCUMBER SUSHI

Cook the sushi rice according to the packet instructions.

Mix together the vinegar and sugar in a bowl and stir until the sugar dissolves.

Once the rice is cooked, while it is still warm, mix in enough of the vinegar-and-sugar mixture to coat the rice grains, but do not allow the rice to become wet. Tip the rice on to a tray to allow it to cool quickly.

Take 1 nori sheet and place it on a bamboo mat with the longest edge parallel to the work surface and the ridged surface facing upwards. With damp hands, cover three-quarters of the nori sheet with a thin layer of rice, leaving a band of nori at the furthest edge from you free of rice. Spread half the wasabi in a line across the front edge of the rice. Place the cucumber strips and half the smoked salmon over the wasabi. Using the bamboo mat, roll up the nori, tucking in the cucumber and salmon as you go. Once you have rolled up the majority of the nori, wet your finger and dampen the clear edge of the nori sheet, then finish rolling up the nori. The wet edge will stick the roll together. Repeat with the remaining nori sheet, wasabi, cucumber and salmon.

Using a sharp knife, cut the rolls into 8 even pieces.

Serve the pickled ginger and soy sauce alongside the nori rolls.

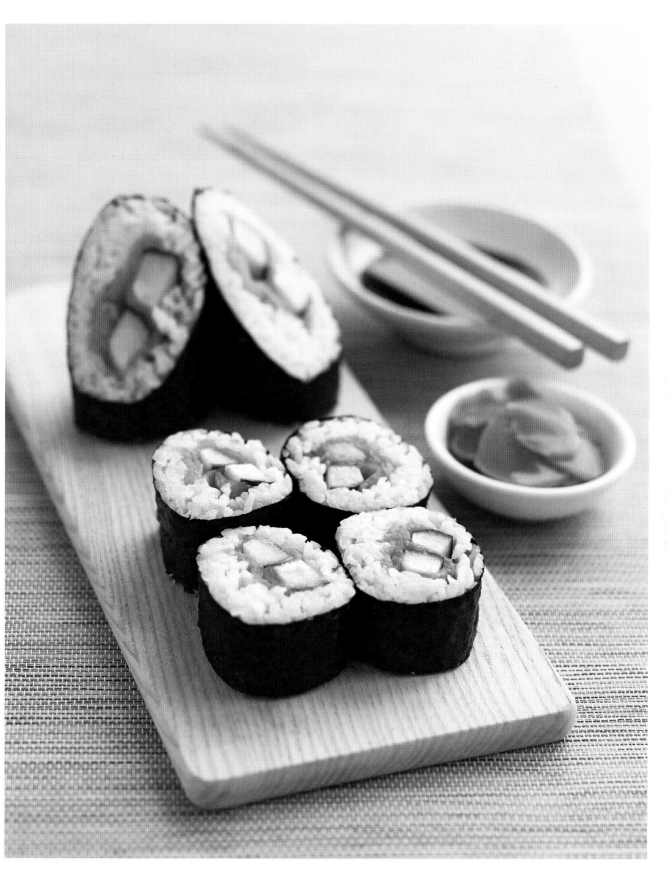

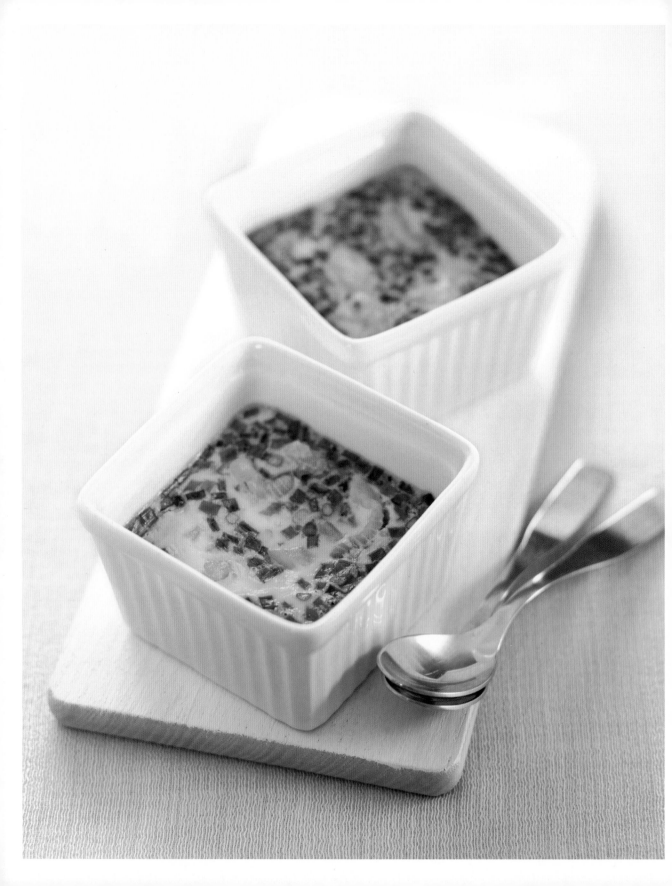

5g (1/8oz) unsalted butter

125g (4 1/2oz) smoked salmon
or smoked trout, cut into
bite-sized pieces

2 large eggs

2 tablespoons cream

1 tablespoon chopped herbs
(such as chervil and chives)

salt and freshly ground
black pepper

toasted gluten-free bread,
to serve (optional)

IT IS A WIDELY
HELD MISCONCEPTION
THAT CREAM CONTAINS
A HIGH LACTOSE LOAD. IT IS,
IN FACT, NATURALLY
RELATIVELY LOW IN LACTOSE
SO IS SUITABLE FOR A
LOW-FODMAP DIET.

BAKED EGGS WITH SALMON

PREPARATION TIME: 5 MINUTES
COOKING TIME: 10 MINUTES
SERVES: 2

Preheat the oven to 200°C (400°F), Gas Mark 6. Grease 2 ramekins, each with a capacity of 150ml (1/4 pint), with the butter. Divide the salmon between the ramekins, then break in the eggs.

Mix together the cream and herbs in a bowl and season to taste with salt and pepper. Pour the seasoned cream into the ramekins and place them in a baking tin.

Half-fill the tin with boiling water, ensuring the water does not reach the rims of the ramekins, and transfer the tin to the oven. Bake for about 10 minutes, until the mixture is just set. Serve with triangles of crunchy fresh toast, if liked.

8 large eggs

1 teaspoon dried oregano

1 tablespoon finely chopped mint

4 tablespoons finely chopped flat-leaf parsley

1 handful of fresh chives, sliced

2 tablespoons olive oil

2 large ripe vine tomatoes, roughly chopped

½ courgette, roughly chopped

100g (3½oz) black olives, pitted

100g (3½oz) feta cheese, crumbled

salt and freshly ground black pepper

crisp green salad, to serve (optional)

GREEK-STYLE SUMMER OMELETTE

PREPARATION TIME: 15 MINUTES
COOKING TIME: 15 MINUTES
SERVES: 4

Whisk the eggs in a bowl and add the oregano, mint, parsley and chives. Season well.

Heat the oil in a large, nonstick ovenproof frying pan. Add the tomatoes, courgette and olives and cook for 3–4 minutes or until the vegetables begin to soften.

Meanwhile, preheat the grill on a medium-high setting.

Reduce the heat under the frying pan to medium and pour the eggs into the frying pan. Cook for 3–4 minutes, stirring as they begin to set, until they are firm but still slightly runny in places.

Scatter over the feta, then place the pan under the grill and cook for 4–5 minutes or until the omelette is puffed up and golden. Cut it into wedges and serve with a crisp green salad, if liked.

PREPARATION TIME: 30 MINUTES, PLUS CHILLING AND COOLING

COOKING TIME: 30–35 MINUTES

MAKES: 6

175g (6oz) rice flour, plus extra for dusting

pinch of salt

100g (3½oz) butter, plus extra for greasing

2 egg yolks

2 teaspoons cold water

FOR THE FILLING

1 tablespoon sunflower oil

4 smoked bacon rashers, about 75g (2¾oz) in total, diced

125g (4½oz) mature Cheddar cheese, grated

3 eggs

200ml (7fl oz) lactose-free or plant-based milk (limit soya to 60ml/4 tablespoons per portion), or standard milk if you know you tolerate lactose

2 teaspoons mustard powder

2 tablespoons chopped chives (optional)

salt and freshly ground black pepper

salad, to serve

THIS DISH MAKES A FANTASTIC LOW-FODMAP BRING-TO-WORK LUNCH, AS IT IS EASILY TRANSPORTABLE AND CAN BE ENJOYED HOT OR COLD.

QUICHES LORRAINE

Preheat the oven to 190°C (375°F), Gas Mark 5. Grease 6 x 10cm (4 inch) individual loose-bottomed fluted tart tins.

For the pastry, put the rice flour, salt and butter into a bowl and rub in with your fingertips until you have fine crumbs. Add the egg yolks and mix to a soft dough, adding the water as required.

Cut the pastry into 6 equal portions, then roll out 1 portion between 2 sheets of clingfilm until it is a little larger than one of the prepared tart tins. Remove the top sheet of clingfilm, turn the pastry over, drape it into the tin and remove the other sheet of clingfilm. Press the pastry into the base and sides of the tin with fingers dusted in rice flour. Trim off the excess pastry a little above the rim of the tin.

Repeat with the remaining pastry portions until 6 tart cases have been made. Place these on a baking sheet and chill for 15 minutes.

Meanwhile, make the filling. Heat the oil in a frying pan. Add the bacon and fry over medium-high heat for 5 minutes, stirring, until golden.

Divide three-quarters of the cheese between the tart cases, then sprinkle the bacon on top.

Beat the eggs, milk and mustard in a jug with a little salt and pepper, then pour the mixture into the tart cases. Sprinkle with the chives, if using, and the remaining cheese. Bake for 25–30 minutes, until the tops are golden and the pastry cases are cooked through. Leave to cool for 5 minutes, then remove from the tins and serve with salad.

850ml (1½ pints)
boiling water

2–3 dried red chillies

2 teaspoons cumin seeds

1 teaspoon coriander seeds

1 teaspoon saffron threads

small bunch of flat-leaf
parsley (use leaves and
stems), plus extra leaves,
torn, to garnish

small bunch of fresh coriander
(use leaves and stems), plus
extra leaves, torn, to garnish

small bunch of mint

4–6 peppercorns

1 teaspoon sea salt

whole chillies, to garnish
(optional)

ALTHOUGH CHILLIES
ARE LOW IN FODMAPS,
SOME PEOPLE FIND THEY
MAKE THEIR DIGESTIVE
SYMPTOMS FLARE UP. OMIT
THE CHILLI IN THIS RECIPE IF
YOU KNOW IT DOESN'T
SUIT YOU.

SIMPLE HERB, CHILLI & SAFFRON BROTH

PREPARATION TIME: 5 MINUTES
COOKING TIME: 10 MINUTES
SERVES: 4

Pour the measured water into a saucepan set over medium heat. Add the remaining ingredients and boil gently for 8–10 minutes.

Strain and discard the herbs. Serve the broth between courses or as a digestive, garnished with herbs and whole chillies, if liked.

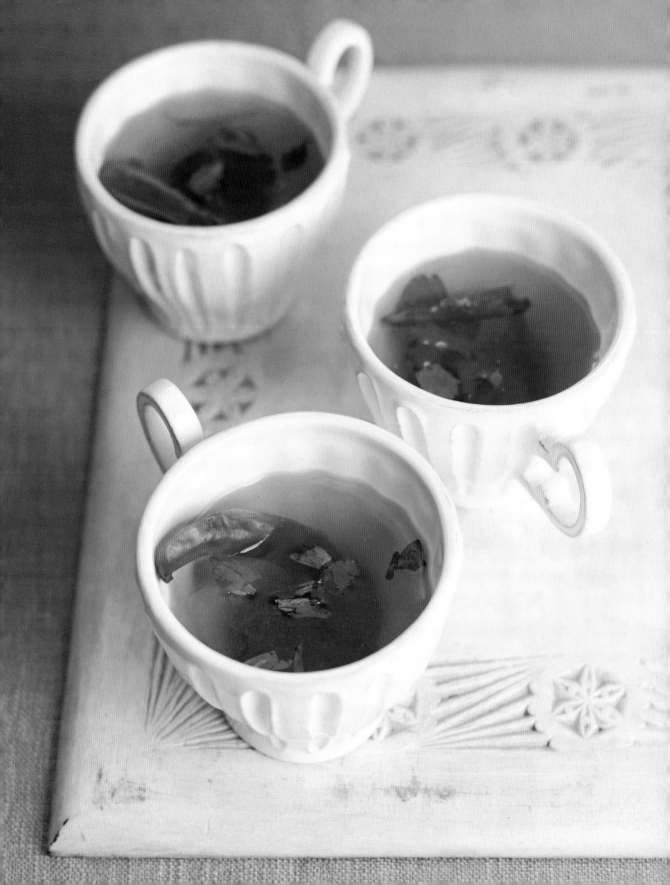

QUICK CHICKEN SOUP

Put the chicken wings, tomatoes, potatoes, spring onions, herbs and spices into a large, heavy-based casserole. Pour over the stock or measured water, add salt to taste and bring to a boil. Cook over medium heat for 25 minutes.

Remove and discard the herbs. Remove and reserve the chicken wings. Strain the vegetables, reserving the stock, and pass them through a food mill or process in a blender until smooth.

Return the blended vegetables, the stock and the chicken wings to the casserole and bring to a boil. Add the rice in a steady stream, stir, and cook over medium heat for a further 5 minutes. Serve immediately.

PREPARATION TIME: 10 MINUTES
COOKING TIME: 30 MINUTES
SERVES: 6

8 chicken wings

3 vine tomatoes

2 potatoes, peeled and halved

1 bunch of spring onions (green parts only), sliced

1 tied bunch of flat-leaf parsley

1 tied bunch of fresh coriander

¼ teaspoon freshly ground black pepper

¼ teaspoon ground turmeric

5 litres (8 pints) low-FODMAP chicken or vegetable stock (*see below*) or water

50g (1¾oz) short-grain rice

salt

LOW-FODMAP VEGETABLE STOCK

Many stocks contain onion and garlic, which should be avoided in a low-FODMAP diet. If you can't find a low-FODMAP version, you might like to make your own using the following recipe.

Heat 2 tablespoons of garlic-infused olive oil in a large saucepan or stockpot. Add 4 large carrots and 2 celery sticks, chopped, cover with a lid and sweat over medium heat for about 10 minutes, until soft. Add 3 litres (5¼ pints) water, followed by 3 bay leaves, 3–4 sprigs of mixed herbs (such as rosemary, thyme, lemon thyme and parsley), a small bunch of chives, 10 peppercorns and a large pinch of salt. Bring to a boil, then gently simmer for 2 hours. Strain the stock. Either use it immediately or leave to cool, then freeze the stock in ice-cube trays and store in the freezer for up to 3 months for readily available low-FODMAP stock.

- 1kg (2lb 4oz) lean stewing beef, diced
- 250g (9oz) boneless lean pork, diced
- 2.5 litres (4½ pints) water
- 24 okra, trimmed and chopped (limit each portion to 60g/2¼oz)
- 500g (1lb 2oz) kale, tough stalks discarded, roughly chopped
- 2 green peppers, deseeded and chopped
- sprig of thyme
- ¼ teaspoon cayenne pepper
- 2 small sweet potatoes, peeled and diced (limit each portion to 70g/2½oz)
- 420g (15oz) potatoes, peeled and sliced
- 2 spring onions (green parts only), roughly chopped
- salt
- gluten-free crusty bread, to serve (optional)

LIMIT OKRA TO 6 PODS PER SERVING TO ENSURE THIS DISH REMAINS LOW-FODMAP-DIET FRIENDLY.

JAMAICAN PEPPER POT SOUP

PREPARATION TIME: 20 MINUTES
COOKING TIME: 1 HOUR 10 MINUTES
SERVES: 6

Put the meat and measured water into a large saucepan. Bring to a boil, then reduce the heat, partially cover the pan with a lid and simmer for about 30 minutes.

Add the okra, kale and green peppers to the saucepan with the thyme and cayenne pepper. Partially cover the pan again and simmer over medium heat for 15 minutes.

Tip in the sweet potatoes, potatoes and spring onions and simmer for a further 20 minutes or until the potatoes are tender and the meat is cooked through. Add more water if the soup is too thick. Season with salt and serve in warmed soup bowls with gluten-free crusty bread, if liked.

100g (3½oz) gluten-free
plain flour

2 teaspoons ground cumin

1 teaspoon chilli powder

2 teaspoons dried oregano

200ml (7fl oz) cold water

400g (14oz) white fish, skinned
and sliced into thick strips

vegetable oil, for deep-frying

salt and freshly ground
black pepper

FOR THE TARTARE SAUCE

100g (3½oz) mayonnaise
(free from garlic and onion)

1 fresh jalapeño chilli,
deseeded, if liked, and
finely chopped

1 teaspoon capers, drained

1 small gherkin (free from
celery seeds), finely chopped

grated zest and juice of
½ lime

handful of fresh coriander
leaves, chopped

TO SERVE

¼ red cabbage

8 gluten-free corn tortillas
(free from pea protein)

FISH TACOS WITH TARTARE SAUCE

PREPARATION TIME: 20 MINUTES
COOKING TIME: 10–15 MINUTES
SERVES: 4

Place the flour, spices, oregano and measured water in a shallow dish and stir together until the mixture resembles thick cream. Season the fish, then dip it in the flour mixture and shake until the fish pieces are well coated.

Fill a large saucepan with the oil to a depth of one-third. Heat to 180–190°C (350–375°F) or until a cube of bread immersed in the oil browns in 15 seconds. Allow any excess coating to fall away from the fish, then deep-fry the fish in batches for 3–5 minutes, until golden and crisp. Remove from the pan, drain on kitchen paper and keep warm.

To make the tartare sauce, mix the mayonnaise, chilli, capers and gherkin in a bowl. Add the lime zest and juice to taste, reserving a dash of lime juice with which to dress the cabbage, then stir in the coriander.

Toss the cabbage with a little salt and the reserved lime juice. Divide the cabbage among the tortillas, then add the deep-fried fish. Drizzle over the tartare sauce and serve immediately.

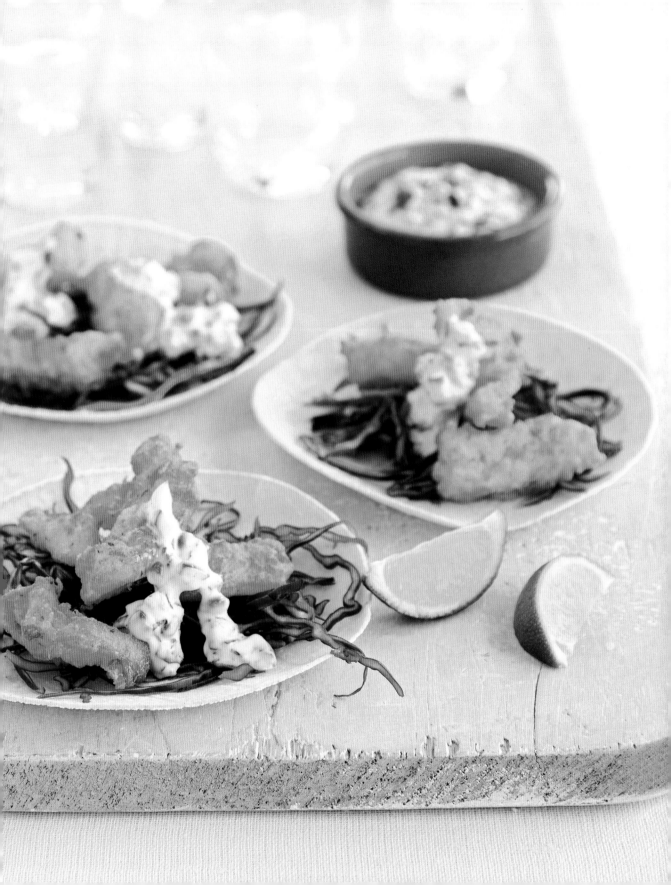

- 2 skinless chicken breasts, halved horizontally
- 2 tablespoons gluten-free plain flour
- 1 egg, beaten
- 125g (4½oz) gluten-free breadcrumbs
- 75g (2¾oz) freshly grated Parmesan cheese
- 3 tablespoons sunflower oil
- 4 small gluten-free bread rolls, split open
- 4 tablespoons mayonnaise (free from garlic and onion)
- 4 small handfuls of green salad leaves
- salt and freshly ground black pepper

CHECK YOUR MAYONNAISE CONTAINS NO HIDDEN ONION OR GARLIC UNDER THE GUISE OF 'FLAVOURINGS'. IF THE LABEL DOES NOT SPECIFY WHICH FLAVOURINGS ARE USED, AVOID THE PRODUCT.

PARMESAN CHICKEN ESCALOPES

PREPARATION TIME: 20 MINUTES
COOKING TIME: 5 MINUTES
SERVES: 4

Place the chicken halves between 2 pieces of clingfilm and beat with a rolling pin to flatten slightly.

Put the flour on to a plate and the beaten egg into a dish. On a separate plate, mix together the breadcrumbs and Parmesan and season with salt and pepper.

Lightly coat each piece of chicken in flour, then shake off any excess flour and dip each piece into the beaten egg. Next, roll it in the breadcrumb mixture to coat, pressing the breadcrumbs on firmly.

Heat the oil in a large frying pan. Add the chicken and cook over medium heat for about 5 minutes, turning once, until golden, crisp and cooked through.

Spread the bread rolls with mayonnaise, then fill with salad leaves and the hot chicken. Serve immediately.

PREPARATION TIME: 25 MINUTES, PLUS COOLING

COOKING TIME: 35 MINUTES

MAKES: 4

1 tablespoon garlic-infused olive oil, plus extra for greasing

1 courgette, diced

1 bunch of spring onions (green parts only), chopped

½ yellow pepper, deseeded and diced

½ red pepper, deseeded and diced

400g (14oz) can chopped tomatoes

1 tablespoon chopped rosemary or basil

½ teaspoon caster sugar

beaten egg, to glaze

salt and freshly ground black pepper

salad, to serve

FOR THE PASTRY

175g (6oz) gluten-free bread flour

75g (2¾oz) butter, diced

75g (2¾oz) mature Cheddar cheese, diced, plus extra, grated, for sprinkling

2 egg yolks

salt and freshly ground black pepper

CHEESY PICNIC PIES

To make the pie filling, heat the oil in a saucepan, add the courgette, spring onions and diced peppers and fry briefly, then add the tomatoes, herbs, sugar and a little salt and pepper. Simmer, uncovered, for 10 minutes, stirring from time to time, until thickened. Leave to cool.

Preheat the oven to 190°C (375°F), Gas Mark 5. Grease a large baking sheet.

To make the pastry, put the flour, butter and a little salt and pepper into a bowl and rub in the butter until the mixture resembles fine breadcrumbs. Stir in the cheese. Add the egg yolks and 2 teaspoons water and mix to form a smooth dough.

Knead the dough lightly, then cut it into 4 pieces. Roll out 1 of the pieces between 2 sheets of clingfilm and pat it into a neat 18cm (7 inch) circle. Remove the top sheet of clingfilm and spoon one-quarter of the filling into the centre of the circle.

Brush the pastry edges with beaten egg, then fold the pastry circle in half, using the lower sheet of clingfilm to help you if necessary. Peel the pastry off the clingfilm, lift it on to the prepared baking sheet, then press the edges together well to seal the pie. Press together any breaks in the pastry. Repeat with the remaining pastry pieces and filling until 4 pies have been made.

Brush the prepared pies with beaten egg, sprinkle with a little extra cheese, then bake for 20 minutes, until golden brown. Transfer the pies to a wire rack. Serve warm or cold with salad.

oil, for greasing

500g (1lb 2oz) good-quality pork sausagemeat

2 teaspoons ground cumin

2 teaspoons ground coriander

2 teaspoons fennel seeds

1 tablespoon ground paprika

1 tablespoon garlic-infused oil

2 spring onions (green parts only), finely chopped

gluten-free flour, for dusting

500g (1lb 2oz) ready-made gluten-free puff pastry

beaten egg, to glaze

salt and freshly ground black pepper

MERGUEZ SAUSAGE ROLLS

PREPARATION TIME: 25 MINUTES
COOKING TIME: 25–30 MINUTES
MAKES: 32

Preheat the oven to 220°C (425°F), Gas Mark 7. Grease a large baking sheet with oil.

Put the sausagemeat into a bowl and add the cumin, coriander, fennel seeds, paprika, garlic-infused oil, spring onions and a little salt and pepper. Mix well with your hands until evenly combined.

Lightly dust your work surface with flour, then roll out the pastry thinly on the floured surface to a 40cm (16 inch) square. Cut the square into 4 strips. Divide the pork mixture into 4 portions and pinch out a portion of the meat mixture along the centre of each strip. Brush the pastry edges with a little beaten egg and fold the pastry strip over the sausagemeat to bring the long edges together. Press the edges of the pastry firmly together to make long, thin logs.

Brush the logs with beaten egg, then cut each log into 8 lengths, each about 5cm (2 inches) long. Transfer the lengths to the prepared baking sheet. Score 2 or 3 cuts along the top of each length using a sharp knife. Bake for 15 minutes, then reduce the oven temperature to 160°C (325°F), Gas Mark 3 and bake for a further 10–15 minutes, until deep golden and cooked through.

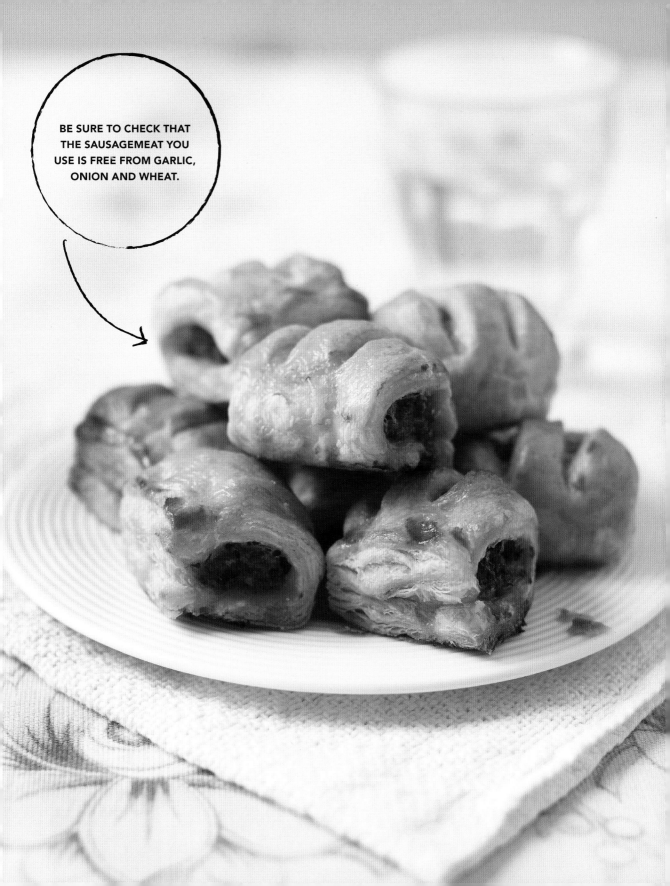

BE SURE TO CHECK THAT THE SAUSAGEMEAT YOU USE IS FREE FROM GARLIC, ONION AND WHEAT.

175g (6oz) gluten-free
plain flour

2 teaspoons gluten-free
baking powder

75g (2¾oz) polenta
or cornmeal

2 tablespoons chopped
flat-leaf parsley

125g (4½oz) mature Cheddar
cheese, finely grated

2 tablespoons capers,
drained and rinsed

1 teaspoon salt

1 teaspoon freshly
ground black pepper

1 large egg

75g (2¾oz) butter, melted

200ml (7fl oz) lactose-free
or plant-based milk (limit
soya to 60ml/4 tablespoons
per portion), or standard
milk if you know you
tolerate lactose

CAPER, CHEESE & POLENTA MUFFINS

PREPARATION TIME: 15 MINUTES, PLUS COOLING
COOKING TIME: 20–25 MINUTES
MAKES: 10

Preheat the oven to 190°C (375°F), Gas Mark 5. Line a 12-hole muffin tin with 10 paper muffin cases.

Sift the flour and baking powder together into a large bowl. Add the polenta or cornmeal, parsley, three-quarters of the cheese, the capers, salt and pepper and mix well.

Beat the egg, melted butter and milk together in a separate bowl. Pour this mixture over the dry ingredients and stir until only just combined – the batter should be lumpy.

Spoon the mixture into the prepared muffin cases so that they are about three-quarters full, then sprinkle the tops with the remaining cheese. Bake for 20–25 minutes, until risen and firm.

Leave to cool in the tin for 5 minutes, then transfer to a wire rack to cool further. Serve warm.

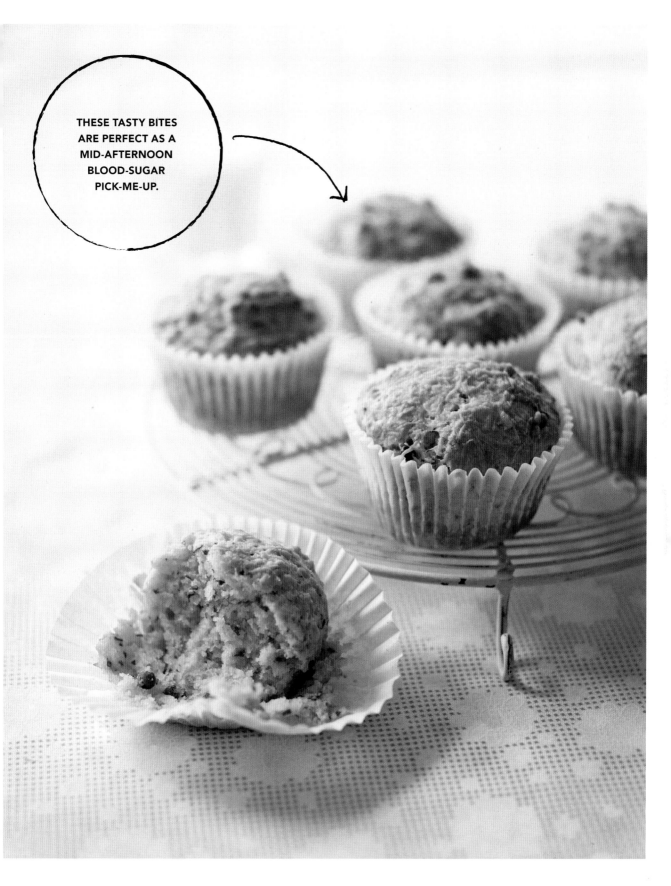

THESE TASTY BITES ARE PERFECT AS A MID-AFTERNOON BLOOD-SUGAR PICK-ME-UP.

200g (7oz) porridge oats

3 sprigs of rosemary, leaves stripped

125g (4½oz) gluten-free plain flour, plus extra for dusting

1 teaspoon gluten-free baking powder

pinch of salt

75g (2¾oz) unsalted butter, cubed

100ml (3½fl oz) lactose-free or plant-based milk (limit soya to 60ml/4 tablespoons per portion), or standard milk if you know you tolerate lactose

lactose-free cheese, to serve

TOP THESE WITH 1 TABLESPOON OF PEANUT OR ALMOND BUTTER, CHEESE, COLD MEATS OR SMOKED SALMON AND CUCUMBER FOR A DELICIOUS SNACK.

HERBED OATCAKES

PREPARATION TIME: 10 MINUTES
COOKING TIME: 15 MINUTES
SERVES: 4

Preheat the oven to 190°C (375°F), Gas Mark 5.

Put the oats and the rosemary leaves into the bowl of a food processor and process until they start to break down and the mixture resembles breadcrumbs.

Add the flour, baking powder and salt and blitz again. Add the butter and process until it is mixed in. Then, with the motor running, pour in the milk and process until the dough comes together in a ball.

Turn out the dough on to a lightly floured work surface and roll it out to a thickness of about 4–5mm (¼ inch). Cut out 20–24 rounds using a 4–5cm (1½–2 inch) cutter, rerolling the dough as necessary.

Arrange the dough rounds on a baking sheet. Bake for 12–15 minutes, until just starting to turn golden at the edges. Cool on a wire rack. Serve with cheese. Store in an airtight container for up to 7 days.

450g (1lb) gluten-free strong white bread flour, plus extra for dusting

....

50g (1¾oz) polenta

....

7g (¼oz) sachet of fast-action dried yeast

....

1 teaspoon salt

....

350ml (12fl oz) warm water

....

5 tablespoons olive oil, plus extra for greasing and brushing

....

1 teaspoon cumin seeds, plus extra to serve

....

1 red chilli, deseeded, if liked, and chopped, plus extra to serve

....

sea salt flakes, to serve (optional)

SPICY GRIDDLED FLATBREADS

PREPARATION TIME: 20 MINUTES, PLUS PROVING
COOKING TIME: 15 MINUTES
MAKES: 8

Place the flour, polenta, yeast and salt in a bowl and mix together. Add the measured water, 3 tablespoons of the oil, the cumin seeds and chilli and mix together to form a dough. Knead the dough using an electric mixer for 5 minutes, or by hand on a lightly floured surface for 10 minutes, until the dough is soft and springy. Put the dough into a lightly oiled bowl, cover with clingfilm and leave to rise in a warm place for about 1 hour, until the mixture has doubled in size.

Tip the dough out on to a lightly floured surface, then punch it down and knead a couple of times until the air is knocked out. Divide the mixture into 8 equal balls and keep loosely covered with lightly oiled clingfilm. Roll out each ball until 5mm (¼ inch) thick.

Heat a griddle pan until smoking hot. Brush the flatbreads with a little oil, then cook, in batches, for 3–5 minutes on each side, until lightly charred and cooked through. Tear the griddled flatbreads into large chunks and serve warm, sprinkled with a little chopped red chilli, some cumin seeds and sea salt flakes, if liked.

SALADS

½ head of white cabbage, thinly sliced

2 carrots, thinly sliced

75g (2¾oz) radishes, thinly sliced

2 spring onions (green parts only), thinly sliced

1 bunch of coriander, chopped

FOR THE DRESSING

1 teaspoon cumin seeds

1 red chilli, deseeded, if liked, and finely chopped

grated zest and juice of 2 limes

2 tablespoons olive oil

salt and freshly ground black pepper

WHILE WHITE AND RED CABBAGE CAN BE ENJOYED ON A LOW-FODMAP DIET, SAVOY CABBAGE NEEDS TO BE LIMITED TO 40G (1½OZ) PER SITTING.

CRUNCHY VEG SALAD

PREPARATION TIME: 10 MINUTES, PLUS STANDING

SERVES: 4

To make the dressing, mix together all the ingredients in a bowl. Season well.

Put the salad ingredients into a serving bowl, add the dressing and toss well. Leave to stand for 5 minutes before serving.

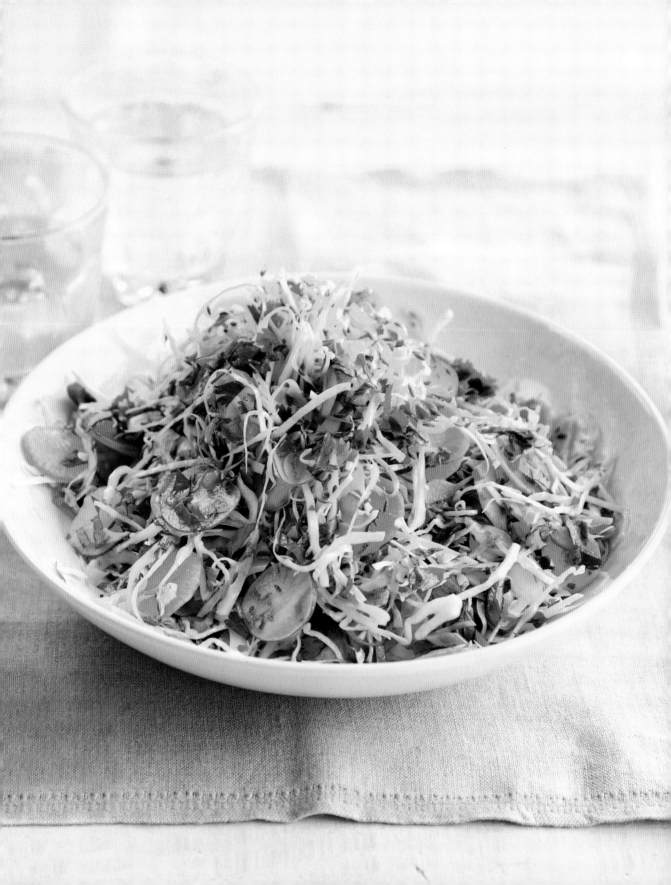

SALMON & WATERCRESS SALAD →

PREPARATION TIME: 10 MINUTES
SERVES: 4

Whisk together the oil, orange juice, mustard and sugar in a small bowl to make a dressing.

In a large bowl, toss together the watercress, cucumber, orange segments and walnuts. Add the smoked salmon and dressing and toss to coat well. Serve with the toasted pitta breads, if liked.

3 tablespoons extra-virgin olive oil

juice of 1 orange

½ teaspoon mustard

½ teaspoon caster sugar

100g (3½oz) watercress

½ cucumber, chopped

2 oranges, peeled and segmented

2 tablespoons toasted walnuts

175g (6oz) smoked salmon strips

4 gluten-free pitta breads, toasted, to serve (optional)

PRAWN & FENNEL SALAD
WITH BASIL CITRUS DRESSING

½ orange

½ lime

handful of snipped chives

25g (1oz) basil leaves

4 tablespoons extra-virgin olive oil

1 fennel bulb, thinly sliced (limit each portion to 50g/1¾oz)

100g (3½oz) green salad leaves

150g (5½oz) cooked peeled large prawns

salt and freshly ground black pepper

PREPARATION TIME: 10 MINUTES
SERVES: 2

Squeeze the juice of the orange and lime into the bowl of a small food processor, add the chives and basil and pulse briefly. With the motor running, slowly add the oil in a thin stream to make a smooth dressing, then season.

Arrange the remaining ingredients on serving plates. Drizzle over the dressing and serve.

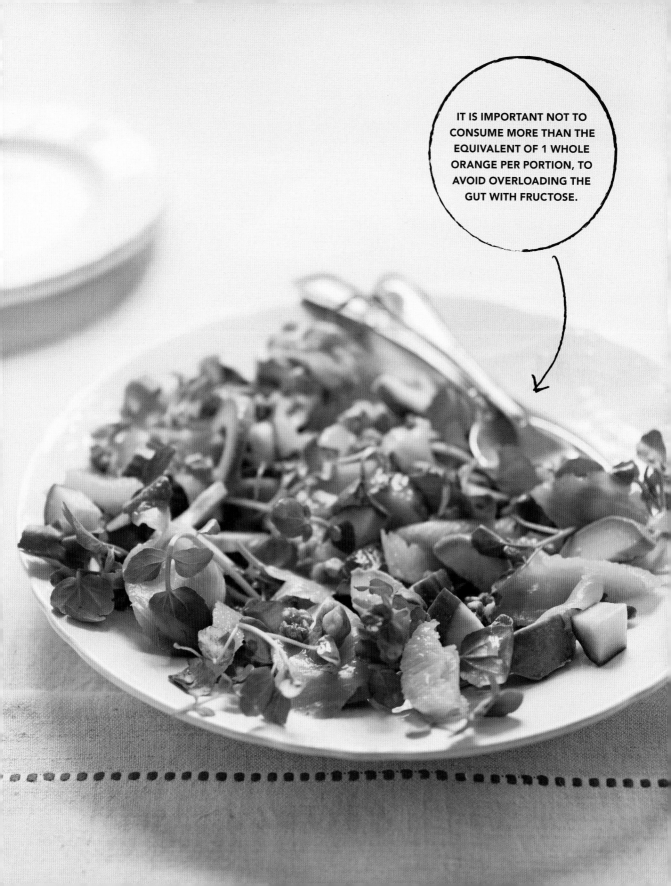

150g (5½oz) quinoa

1 small yellow pepper, deseeded and diced

1 small red pepper, deseeded and diced

4 spring onions (green parts only), sliced

⅓ cucumber, deseeded and diced

½ fennel bulb, finely diced

2 tablespoons finely chopped curly parsley

2 tablespoons finely chopped mint

2 tablespoons finely chopped fresh coriander

2 tablespoons sunflower seeds

finely grated zest and juice of 2 limes

FOR THE DRESSING

4 teaspoons Low-FODMAP Harissa Paste (*see page 128*)

finely grated zest and juice of 2 limes

8 tablespoons sunflower oil

salt and freshly ground black pepper

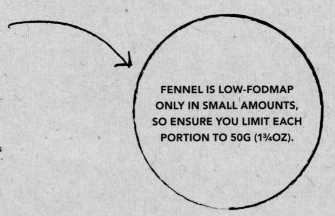

FENNEL IS LOW-FODMAP ONLY IN SMALL AMOUNTS, SO ENSURE YOU LIMIT EACH PORTION TO 50G (1¾OZ).

ZESTY QUINOA SALAD

PREPARATION TIME: 15 MINUTES
COOKING TIME: 15–20 MINUTES
SERVES: 4

Put the quinoa into a saucepan of cold water, bring to a boil and cook for 15–20 minutes or until the quinoa is translucent and just cooked. Drain and rinse thoroughly in cold water.

Meanwhile, make the dressing. Put the harissa paste, lime zest and juice and oil into a bowl or jug and whisk well to blend. Season to taste and set aside.

Mix the quinoa in a large bowl with the prepared vegetables and herbs, 1 tablespoon of the sunflower seeds and the lime juice and zest. Scatter over the remaining sunflower seeds and serve with the dressing.

MIDDLE-EASTERN BREAD SALAD

**PREPARATION TIME: 10 MINUTES,
  PLUS COOLING**

COOKING TIME: 2–3 MINUTES

SERVES: 4–6

2 gluten-free flatbreads or
gluten-free soft tortillas

1 large green pepper, deseeded
and diced

1 small Lebanese cucumber
or ¼ regular cucumber, diced

250g (9oz) cherry tomatoes,
halved

1 handful of chives, finely
snipped

2 tablespoons chopped mint

2 tablespoons chopped flat-leaf
parsley

2 tablespoons chopped fresh
coriander

3 tablespoons olive oil

4 tablespoons lemon juice

salt and freshly ground black
pepper

Toast the flatbreads or tortillas on a preheated griddle pan or under a preheated hot grill for 2–3 minutes or until charred. Leave to cool, then tear into bite-sized pieces.

Put the green pepper, cucumber, tomatoes and herbs into a serving bowl. Add the oil and lemon juice, season with salt and pepper and toss well. Add the bread and stir again. Serve immediately.

200g (7oz) vermicelli rice noodles

½ cucumber, deseeded and cut into matchsticks

1 carrot, cut into matchsticks

150g (5½oz) bean sprouts

125g (4½oz) green beans, cut into thin strips

2 tablespoons chopped fresh coriander

2 tablespoons chopped mint

1 red chilli, deseeded and thinly sliced

2 tablespoons chopped blanched peanuts, to garnish

FOR THE DRESSING

1 tablespoon sunflower or groundnut oil

½ teaspoon caster sugar

1 tablespoon Thai fish sauce

2 tablespoons freshly squeezed lime juice

VIETNAMESE-STYLE VEGETABLE NOODLE SALAD

PREPARATION TIME: 20 MINUTES
COOKING TIME: 5 MINUTES
SERVES: 4

Bring a large saucepan of water to a boil, then turn off the heat and add the rice noodles. Cover and leave to cook for 4 minutes, until just tender (alternatively, cook according to the packet instructions). Drain the noodles and cool immediately in a bowl of ice-cold water.

To make the dressing, put the ingredients into a small bowl and stir until the sugar is dissolved.

Place the prepared vegetables, herbs and chilli in a large mixing bowl. Pour over half of the dressing and toss until well combined.

Drain the noodles and transfer to four serving bowls. Heap the salad on top of the noodles and drizzle with the remaining dressing. Serve scattered with chopped peanuts.

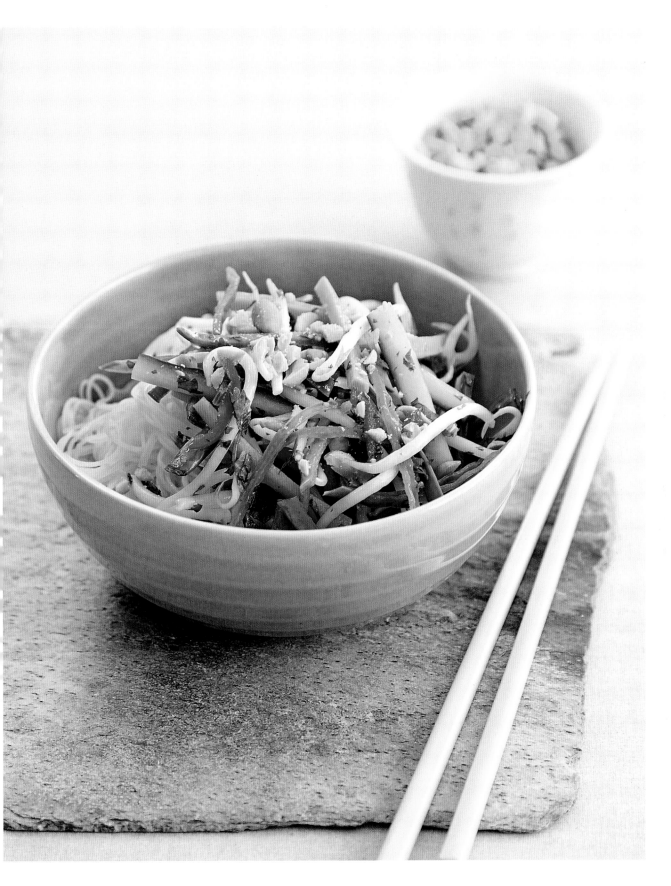

250g (9oz) cherry tomatoes, halved

1 tablespoon olive oil

150g (5½oz) mini mozzarella cheese balls, drained

25g (1oz) pine nuts, toasted

sea salt and freshly ground black pepper

gluten-free bread, to serve

FOR THE DRESSING

25g (1oz) rocket leaves

12 basil leaves

4 tablespoons extra-virgin olive oil

1 teaspoon red wine vinegar

sea salt and freshly ground black pepper

ROAST TOMATO & MOZZARELLA SALAD

PREPARATION TIME: 10 MINUTES, PLUS COOLING
COOKING TIME: 20 MINUTES
SERVES: 4

Preheat the oven to 200°C (400°F), Gas Mark 6.

Place the tomatoes with their cut sides facing up in a small roasting tin. Drizzle over the olive oil and season with a little sea salt and pepper. Roast for 20 minutes, until softened. Remove the tomatoes from the oven and leave to cool.

To make the dressing, put the rocket and basil leaves, 2 tablespoons of the extra-virgin olive oil and the vinegar into a small bowl and blend with a stick blender to a purée (alternatively, blend the mixture using a mini food processor). Stir in the remaining oil and season to taste with salt and pepper.

Arrange the roasted tomatoes on a platter, then tear the mozzarella balls in half and arrange the mozzarella chunks among the tomatoes. Drizzle over the dressing and scatter over the pine nuts. Serve immediately with gluten-free bread.

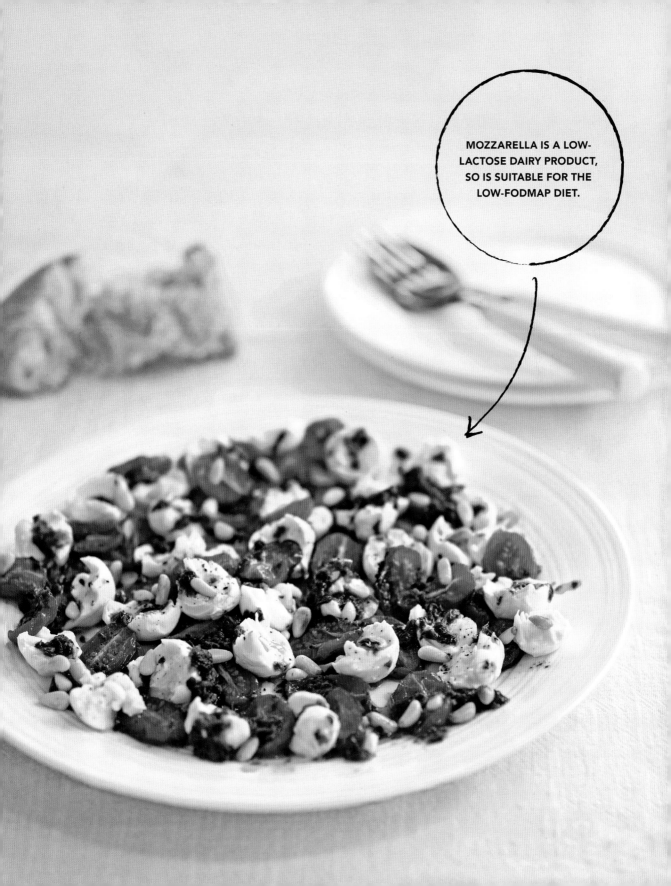

MOZZARELLA IS A LOW-LACTOSE DAIRY PRODUCT, SO IS SUITABLE FOR THE LOW-FODMAP DIET.

400g (14oz) white crabmeat

1 large orange, peeled and sliced

50g (1¾oz) rocket

1 bunch of spring onions (green parts only), sliced

200g (7oz) steamed green beans, sliced

salt and freshly ground black pepper

FOR THE WATERCRESS DRESSING

85g (3oz) watercress, tough stems removed

1 tablespoon Dijon mustard

2 tablespoons olive oil

salt

TO SERVE

4 gluten-free pitta breads

lime wedges

CRAB & ORANGE SALAD

PREPARATION TIME: 15 MINUTES
COOKING TIME: 2 MINUTES
SERVES: 4

Combine the crabmeat, orange, rocket, spring onions and green beans in a serving dish. Season to taste with salt and pepper.

To make the dressing, put the watercress, mustard and oil into the bowl of a food processor and blend together. Season with salt.

Toast the pitta breads. Stir the dressing into the salad and serve with the toasted pitta breads and lime wedges on the side.

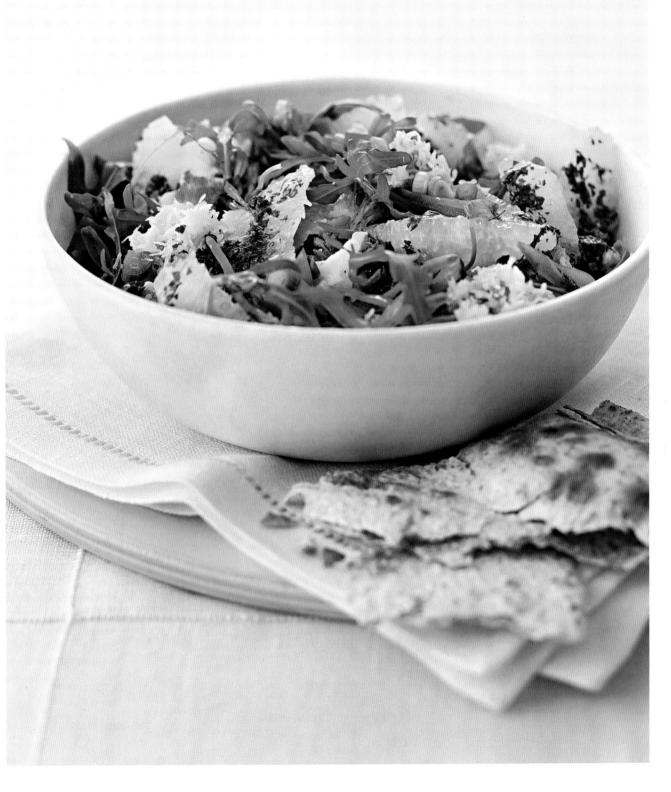

400g (14oz) waxy new potatoes,
halved
....

3 tablespoons olive oil
....

2 teaspoons red wine vinegar
....

1 tablespoon wholegrain
mustard
....

1 handful of chives, finely
snipped
....

1 tablespoon rinsed and thinly
sliced cornichons or gherkins
(free from celery seeds)
....

2 teaspoons rinsed and drained
capers
....

125g (4½oz) cherry tomatoes,
halved
....

2 tablespoons Kalamata olives,
drained
....

4 small mackerel fillets,
boned and skins lightly scored
....

large handful of frisée
lettuce leaves
....

salt and freshly ground
black pepper

WARM POTATO
& MACKEREL SALAD

PREPARATION TIME: 15 MINUTES,
   PLUS COOLING
COOKING TIME: 20 MINUTES
SERVES: 4

Cook the new potatoes in a large pan of salted boiling water for
12–15 minutes, until just tender. Drain the potatoes, return them to
the pan and toss with 2 tablespoons of the olive oil. Add the vinegar,
mustard, chives, cornichons or gherkins, capers, tomatoes and olives,
then season to taste. Set aside.

Heat the remaining olive oil in a large, nonstick frying pan and cook
the mackerel fillets, with their skin sides facing down, for 3–4 minutes,
until the flesh turns white. Gently turn them over and cook for a further
minute, until lightly golden. Remove from the pan and leave to cool
slightly, then flake the flesh.

Arrange the frisée on serving plates and serve with the warm potato
salad and flaked mackerel.

2 teaspoons garlic-infused olive oil

1 teaspoon balsamic vinegar

4 small boneless, skinless chicken breasts, halved horizontally

FOR THE RICE SALAD

200g (7oz) mixture of wild rice and basmati rice

2 red peppers, roasted, deseeded and sliced

3 spring onions (green parts only), sliced

125g (4½oz) cherry tomatoes, quartered

75g (2¾oz) rocket leaves

75g (2¾oz) lactose-free soft goats' cheese, crumbled

FOR THE DRESSING

2 tablespoons lemon juice

1 teaspoon Dijon mustard

1 teaspoon maple syrup

2 tablespoons olive oil

WILD RICE & GRIDDLED CHICKEN SALAD

PREPARATION TIME: 40 MINUTES, PLUS MARINATING
COOKING TIME: 35 MINUTES
SERVES: 4

Mix together the garlic-infused oil and vinegar in a non-metallic bowl, add the chicken and coat in the marinade. Cover and leave to marinate in the refrigerator for at least 30 minutes.

Cook the rice in a saucepan of boiling water according to the packet instructions. Drain well and leave to cool, then mix with the peppers, spring onions, tomatoes, rocket and goats' cheese in a large bowl.

Whisk together the dressing ingredients in a bowl. Stir the dressing into the rice salad. Spoon the salad on to 4 serving plates.

Heat a griddle pan until hot. Cook the chicken over medium-high heat for 3–4 minutes on each side, until cooked through. Immediately before serving, slice the griddled chicken and arrange it on top of the salad.

4 tablespoons olive oil

750g (1lb 10oz) butternut squash, peeled, if liked, deseeded and cut into small chunks

380g (13oz) chicken livers

175g (6oz) bacon, cut into strips

100g (3½oz) walnuts

160g (5½oz) watercress

freshly ground black pepper

balsamic vinegar, to serve

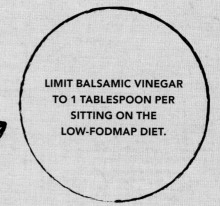

LIMIT BALSAMIC VINEGAR TO 1 TABLESPOON PER SITTING ON THE LOW-FODMAP DIET.

WARM CHICKEN LIVER, BUTTERNUT SQUASH & BACON SALAD

PREPARATION TIME: 10 MINUTES, PLUS COOLING
COOKING TIME: 20 MINUTES
SERVES: 4

Heat 3 tablespoons of the oil in a large, heavy-based frying pan or wok and cook the squash, stirring occasionally, over medium-high heat for 15–20 minutes, until softened and cooked through.

Meanwhile, in a separate heavy-based frying pan, heat the remaining oil and cook the chicken livers and bacon over high heat for 10 minutes or until golden and cooked through, stirring almost continuously to prevent sticking. Add the walnuts and cook for a further minute to warm through.

Toss together the chicken livers, bacon, walnuts and squash in a large bowl, season with pepper and set aside to cool for 3–4 minutes.

Just before serving, add the watercress to the bowl and toss to mix. Arrange the salad on 4 warmed serving plates and drizzle with balsamic vinegar.

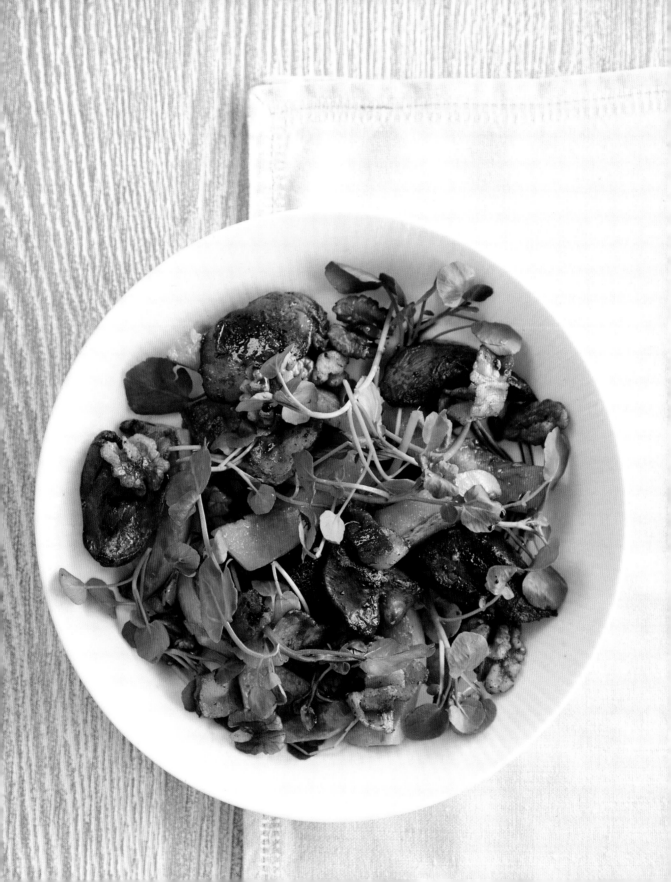

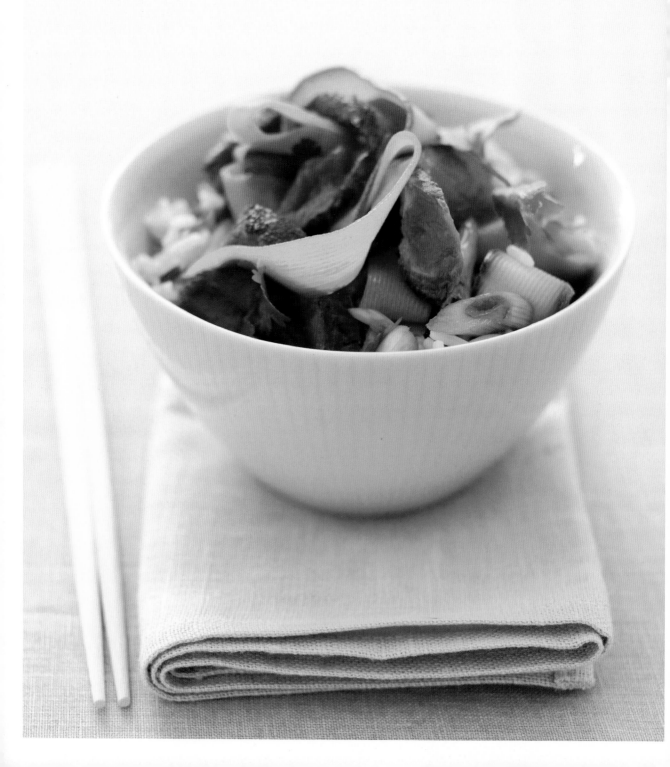

MARINATED THAI BEEF SALAD

PREPARATION TIME: 25 MINUTES
COOKING TIME: 20–25 MINUTES
SERVES: 4

150g (5½oz) mixture of long-grain rice and wild rice

finely grated zest and juice of 2 limes

700g (1lb 9oz) thick-cut sirloin steak or rump steak

2 tablespoons sesame oil

2 courgettes, cut into long, thin slices with a vegetable peeler

2 carrots, cut into long, thin slices with a vegetable peeler

4 spring onions (green parts only), thinly sliced

1 large mild red chilli, deseeded and chopped

4cm (1½ inch) piece of fresh root ginger, peeled and cut into thin strips

2 tablespoons soy sauce

4 tablespoons dry sherry or water

1 tablespoon Thai fish sauce

2 teaspoons caster sugar

small bunch of fresh coriander or mint, roughly torn

Cook the rice in a saucepan of boiling water for 15–18 minutes or until just tender. Drain the cooked rice, rinse it in cold water, then drain thoroughly. Put the rice into a bowl with the lime zest and juice and toss together. Cover the bowl and place in the refrigerator.

Heat a frying pan over high heat. Brush the steaks with the sesame oil, then cook them in the hot frying pan over high heat for 1–3 minutes on each side, depending on your preference. Transfer to a shallow non-metallic dish.

Put the courgette and carrot strips into the hot frying pan you used to cook the steaks. Add the spring onions, chilli and ginger and fry briefly for 30 seconds. Transfer to the dish with the steak. Add the soy sauce, sherry or water, fish sauce and sugar to the pan and warm gently. Pour the mixture over the steak and vegetables and leave to marinate and cool, then chill until required.

When ready to serve, transfer the rice to a salad bowl. Add the vegetables and sauce and the torn herbs and toss to combine. Cut the steak into thin slices and arrange on top of the rice salad.

5 tablespoons extra-virgin olive oil

400g (14oz) very fresh tuna steak

1 tablespoon black peppercorns, coarsely crushed

1 tablespoon balsamic vinegar

100g (3½oz) wild rocket leaves

salt

shavings of Parmesan cheese, to serve

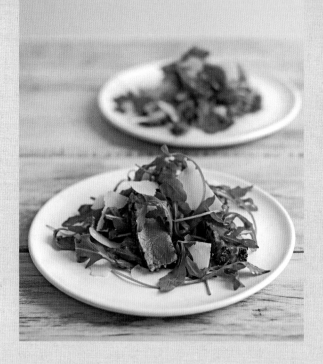

PEPPERED TUNA
WITH ROCKET & PARMESAN

PREPARATION TIME: 10 MINUTES, PLUS COOLING
COOKING TIME: 10 MINUTES
SERVES: 4

Brush 1 tablespoon of the oil over the tuna. Place the crushed peppercorns on a plate, then roll the tuna in the pepper until well coated. Wrap up the tuna tightly in a piece of kitchen foil.

Heat a dry, heavy-based frying pan until smoking hot. Add the wrapped tuna to the pan and cook for 7 minutes, turning every minute or so to cook evenly on each side. Remove from the pan and leave to cool a little.

Whisk the remaining oil with the vinegar until well combined, then season with salt.

Just before serving, unwrap the tuna and slice it. Toss the rocket with the dressing and arrange it on serving plates. Scatter over the tuna and sprinkle with Parmesan shavings to serve.

400g (14oz) gluten-free pasta

150g (5½oz) green beans, trimmed

200g (7oz) can tuna in spring water, drained and flaked

100g (3½oz) cherry tomatoes, quartered

50g (1¾oz) pitted black olives

75g (2¾oz) rocket

salt

FOR THE DRESSING

3 anchovy fillets in oil, drained and chopped

2 teaspoons white wine vinegar

2 tablespoons garlic-infused olive oil

ENSURE THAT GARLIC-INFUSED OIL IS STRAINED WELL AND CONTAINS NO VISIBLE GARLIC RESIDUE.

PASTA NIÇOISE

PREPARATION TIME: 10 MINUTES
COOKING TIME: 10 MINUTES
SERVES: 4

Cook the pasta in a large saucepan of salted boiling water according to the packet instructions until al dente, adding the beans 5 minutes before the end of the cooking time and cooking until the beans are just tender.

Meanwhile, make the dressing. Mash the anchovies in a bowl, then mix in the vinegar and oils.

Drain the pasta and beans, reserving a little of the cooking water. Return the mixture to the pan and stir through the dressing, adding just enough of the reserved cooking water to loosen, if needed. Mix through the remaining ingredients and serve immediately.

8 slices of day-old gluten-free bread, cut into bite-sized pieces

6 tablespoons olive oil

4 eggs

1 tablespoon Dijon mustard

2 tablespoons lemon juice

100g (3½oz) bacon, cut into bite-sized pieces

100g (3½oz) rocket leaves

salt and freshly ground black pepper

MOST MUSTARD IS SUITABLE FOR THE LOW-FODMAP DIET, BUT READ THE LABEL TO DOUBLE-CHECK IT DOES NOT CONTAIN ONION, GARLIC OR FRUCTOSE.

SOFT-BOILED EGG & BACON SALAD

PREPARATION TIME: 10 MINUTES
COOKING TIME: 10 MINUTES
SERVES: 4

Preheat the oven to 200°C (400°F), Gas Mark 6.

Put the bread into a bowl, add 2 tablespoons of the oil and toss to coat. Spread out the pieces of bread on a baking sheet and bake for 10 minutes or until golden brown.

Meanwhile, cook the eggs in a saucepan of boiling water for 4 minutes. Drain, then cool them under cold running water for 1 minute.

Whisk together the remaining oil, the mustard and lemon juice in a small bowl.

Heat a nonstick frying pan, add the bacon and cook over medium heat for 5 minutes, until crisp and golden. Put the bacon pieces into a bowl with the rocket.

Shell the eggs, then break them in half and add them to the bacon and rocket. Scatter over the croûtons, then drizzle over the dressing. Season to taste and serve immediately.

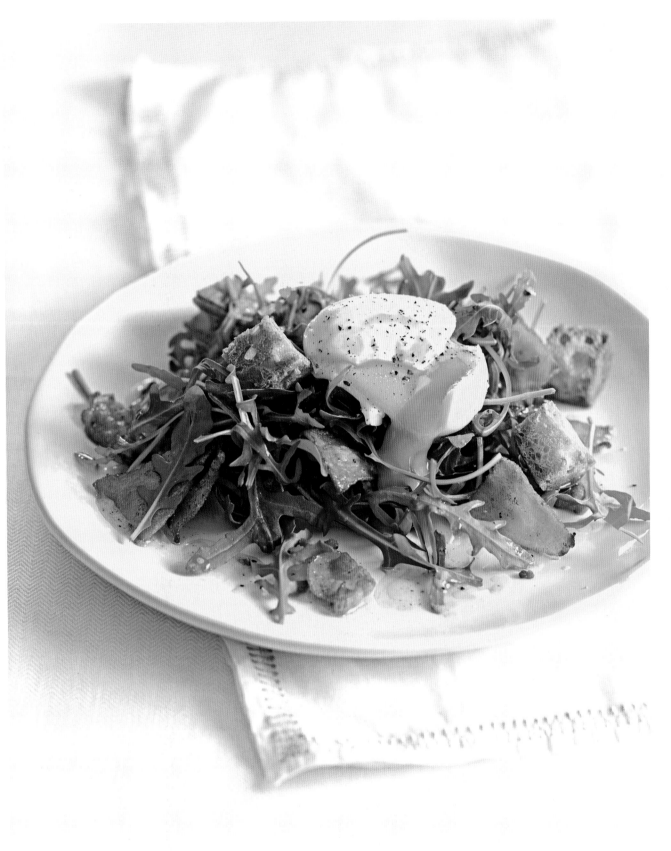

STARTERS & LIGHT BITES

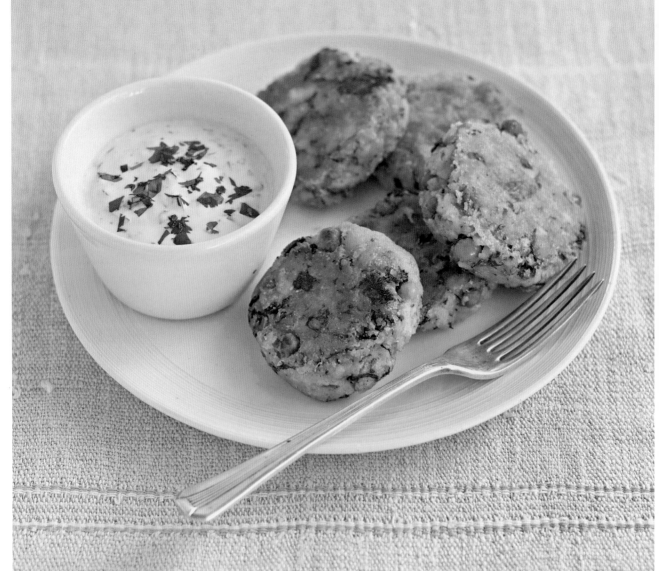

WHEN USING GARAM MASALA, CHECK TO ENSURE YOUR PRODUCT DOES NOT CONTAIN FODMAPS SUCH AS ONION AND GARLIC.

750g (1lb 10oz) potatoes, peeled and cut into chunks

2 tablespoons chopped fresh coriander

2 teaspoons peeled and finely grated fresh root ginger

2½ teaspoons garam masala

1 mild green chilli, deseeded and chopped

100g (3½oz) frozen spinach, defrosted

75g (2¾oz) fresh gluten-free breadcrumbs

2–3 tablespoons gluten-free plain flour

vegetable oil, for shallow-frying

salt and freshly ground black pepper

FOR THE CHUTNEY

2 tablespoons chopped fresh coriander

2 tablespoons chopped mint

200ml (7fl oz) plain lactose-free or plant-based yogurt (limit soya yogurt to 60g/2¼oz per portion), or standard yogurt if you know you tolerate lactose

2 teaspoons lemon juice

salt and freshly ground black pepper

ALOO TIKKI
WITH CORIANDER & MINT CHUTNEY

PREPARATION TIME: 20 MINUTES
COOKING TIME: 25 MINUTES
SERVES: 4

Cook the potatoes in a large saucepan of lightly salted boiling water for about 10 minutes or until just tender. Drain well.

Meanwhile, mix the coriander with the grated ginger, garam masala and chopped chilli in a bowl.

Place the spinach in the middle of a clean tea towel, bring up the edges and twist the spinach in the tea towel over a sink to squeeze out excess moisture. Add to the bowl of spices, season generously with salt and pepper and mix well to combine. Set aside.

To make the chutney, mix the coriander with the mint, yogurt and lemon juice. Season to taste, then set aside.

Add the potatoes to the spinach and mash well to combine. Add the breadcrumbs and mix thoroughly to form a soft dough mixture. Form the mixture into 20–24 small patties and dust with the flour.

Heat the oil in a large frying pan. Shallow-fry the patties over medium heat for 3–4 minutes, turning once, until crisp and golden. Drain on kitchen paper, then serve hot with the chutney.

PREPARATION TIME: 20 MINUTES
COOKING TIME: 20 MINUTES
SERVES: 4

450g (1lb) potatoes, peeled and diced

3 tablespoons olive oil

500g (1lb 2oz) skinless salmon fillet

1 tablespoon chopped dill

finely grated zest of 1 lemon

gluten-free plain flour, for dusting

1 egg, beaten

75g (2¾/oz) dried gluten-free breadcrumbs

salt and freshly ground black pepper

green salad, to serve

FOR THE DILL SAUCE

3 tablespoons mayonnaise (free from garlic and onion)

3 tablespoons plain lactose-free or plant-based yogurt (limit soya yogurt to 60g/2¼oz per portion), or standard yogurt if you know you tolerate lactose

handful of dill, chopped

1 cornichon, sliced

SALMON FISHCAKES
WITH DILL SAUCE

Preheat the grill on the highest setting.

Cook the potatoes in a saucepan of lightly salted boiling water for 12 minutes, until soft. Drain well and roughly mash.

Meanwhile, rub 1 teaspoon of the oil over the salmon and season well. Transfer to a baking tray and grill for 10 minutes, until cooked through. Leave to cool a little, then break the flesh into large flakes.

Combine the sauce ingredients in a bowl and mix well.

Mix together the mashed potato, salmon flakes, dill and lemon zest in a large bowl. Lightly wet your hands, then shape the mixture into 8 fishcakes. Dust each fishcake with a little flour, dip it into the egg and, finally, dip it into the breadcrumbs until well coated.

Heat the remaining oil in a large, nonstick frying pan. Cook the fishcakes for 3–4 minutes on each side, until golden and crisp. Serve with a green salad and the dill sauce.

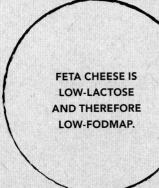

FETA CHEESE IS
LOW-LACTOSE
AND THEREFORE
LOW-FODMAP.

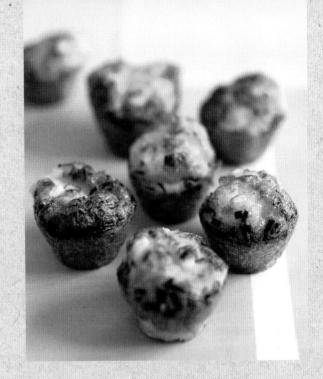

MINI TOMATO & FETA OMELETTES

PREPARATION TIME: 10 MINUTES

COOKING TIME: 10 MINUTES

MAKES: 12

rapeseed or vegetable oil,
for greasing

4 eggs, beaten

2 tablespoons chopped chives

3 sun-dried tomatoes, finely
sliced

75g (2¾oz) feta cheese,
crumbled

salt and freshly ground black
pepper

Preheat the oven to 220°C (425°F), Gas Mark 7. Lightly grease
a 12-hole mini muffin tin with oil.

Mix together all the ingredients in a large bowl until just combined.
Pour the mixture into the prepared recesses of the muffin tin.

Bake for about 10 minutes, until golden and puffed up. Transfer
to a wire rack and leave to cool a little. Serve warm.

½ tablespoon rapeseed oil

400g (14oz) baby spinach leaves

6 large eggs

100ml (3½fl oz) lactose-free or plant-based milk (limit soya to 60ml/4 tablespoons per portion), or standard milk if you know you tolerate lactose

3 tablespoons grated Parmesan cheese

2 tablespoons finely chopped chives

150g (5½oz) cooked hot-smoked trout or salmon fillets, flaked

4 cherry tomatoes, halved

salt and freshly ground black pepper

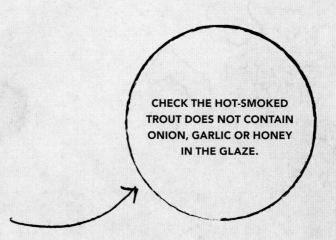

CHECK THE HOT-SMOKED TROUT DOES NOT CONTAIN ONION, GARLIC OR HONEY IN THE GLAZE.

MINI SMOKED TROUT QUICHES

PREPARATION TIME: 15 MINUTES, PLUS COOLING

COOKING TIME: 20 MINUTES

SERVES: 4

Preheat the oven to 180°C (350°F), Gas Mark 4. Line 8 holes of a muffin tin with 15cm (6 inch) squares of greaseproof paper.

Heat the oil in a frying pan, add the spinach and cook briefly until wilted. Remove the pan from the heat.

Beat together the eggs, milk and cheese in a jug and season to taste, then stir in the chives and trout or salmon.

Divide the spinach between the muffin cases, then pour in the egg mixture. Top each one with a tomato half. Bake for 12–15 minutes, until just set. Transfer to a wire rack and leave to cool a little. Serve warm or cold.

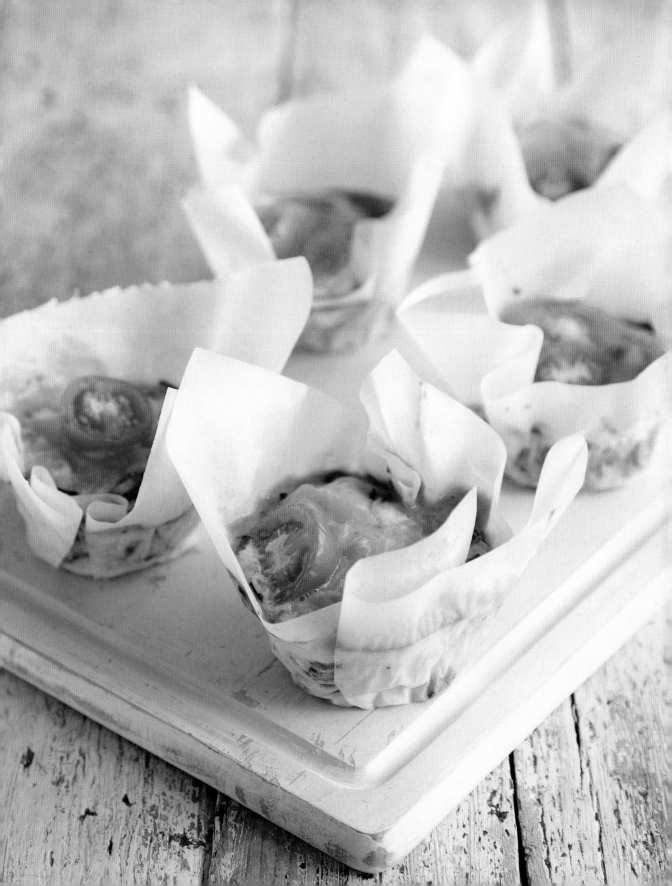

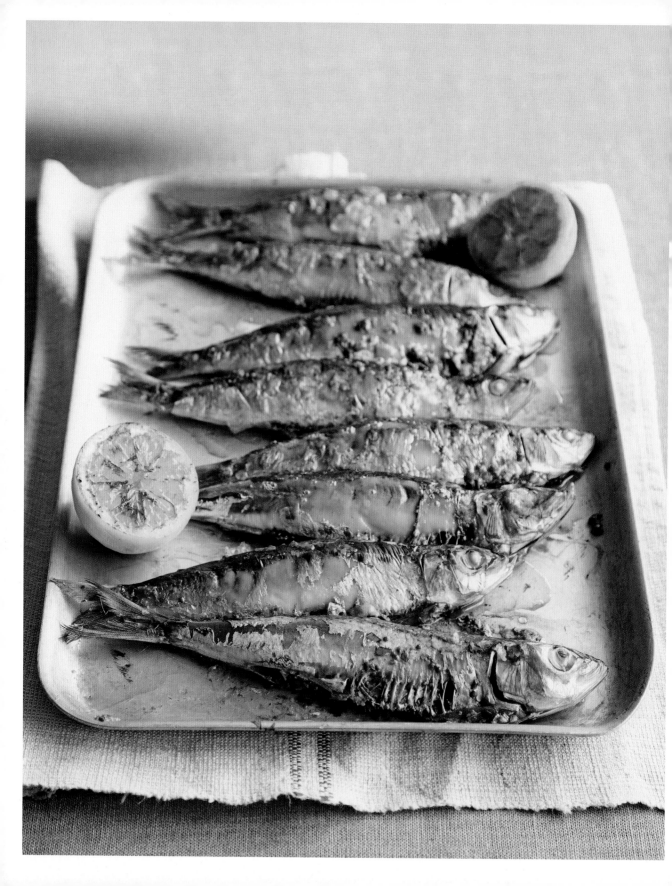

small handful of flat-leaf
parsley leaves, chopped

1 tablespoon wholegrain
mustard

4 tablespoons lemon juice

8 sardines, boned, cleaned
and gutted

2 tablespoons olive oil

lemon halves, to serve

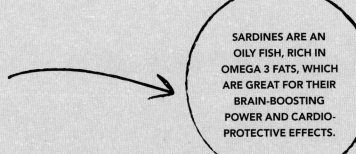

SARDINES ARE AN
OILY FISH, RICH IN
OMEGA 3 FATS, WHICH
ARE GREAT FOR THEIR
BRAIN-BOOSTING
POWER AND CARDIO-
PROTECTIVE EFFECTS.

GRILLED LEMON &
MUSTARD SARDINES

PREPARATION TIME: 15 MINUTES
COOKING TIME: 10 MINUTES
SERVES: 4

Preheat the grill on the highest setting.

Mix together the parsley, mustard and lemon juice in a bowl, then spoon the mixture into the sardine cavities. Brush the fish with the oil.

Cook under the hot grill for 4 minutes on each side or until cooked through. Serve with lemon halves.

PREPARATION TIME:
25 MINUTES, PLUS SOAKING
AND MARINATING
COOKING TIME: 25 MINUTES
SERVES: 4

3 dried ancho chillies, trimmed and deseeded

3 cloves

½ teaspoon cumin seeds

½ cinnamon stick

2 teaspoons dried oregano

1 tablespoon red wine vinegar

2 teaspoons maple syrup

1 tablespoon garlic-infused olive oil

2 small pork tenderloins, about 300g (10½oz) each (or 1 large tenderloin, about 450g/1lb)

salt and freshly ground black pepper

FOR THE SALSA

½ ripe pineapple, peeled, cored and chopped

1 tablespoon finely chopped spring onions (green parts only)

1 red chilli, deseeded, if liked, and chopped

juice of ½ lime

handful of fresh coriander leaves, chopped

salt and freshly ground black pepper

SPICED PORK WITH PINEAPPLE SALSA

Heat a dry nonstick frying pan until hot. Add the chillies and dry-fry for 1 minute on each side, until lightly toasted. Transfer to a heatproof bowl, pour over enough boiling water to cover and leave to soak for 30 minutes, until softened.

Add the whole spices to the same frying pan you used to cook the chillies and cook for 30 seconds, until they release their aromas. Tip the mixture into a spice grinder (or use a pestle and mortar) and grind until finely ground.

Remove the chillies from the soaking liquid and put them into a mini processor or blender with the ground spices, oregano, vinegar, maple syrup and oil and whizz to a smooth paste. Rub the mixture all over the pork in a shallow non-metallic dish, cover the dish with clingfilm and leave to marinate in the refrigerator for 2 hours.

Preheat the oven to 200°C (400°F), Gas Mark 6.

Wipe away any excess marinade from the pork, then place it in a shallow baking tray and season. Bake for 25 minutes, until just cooked through.

Meanwhile, make the salsa. Combine all the ingredients in a bowl. Season and mix well.

Cut the pork into thick slices and serve with the salsa.

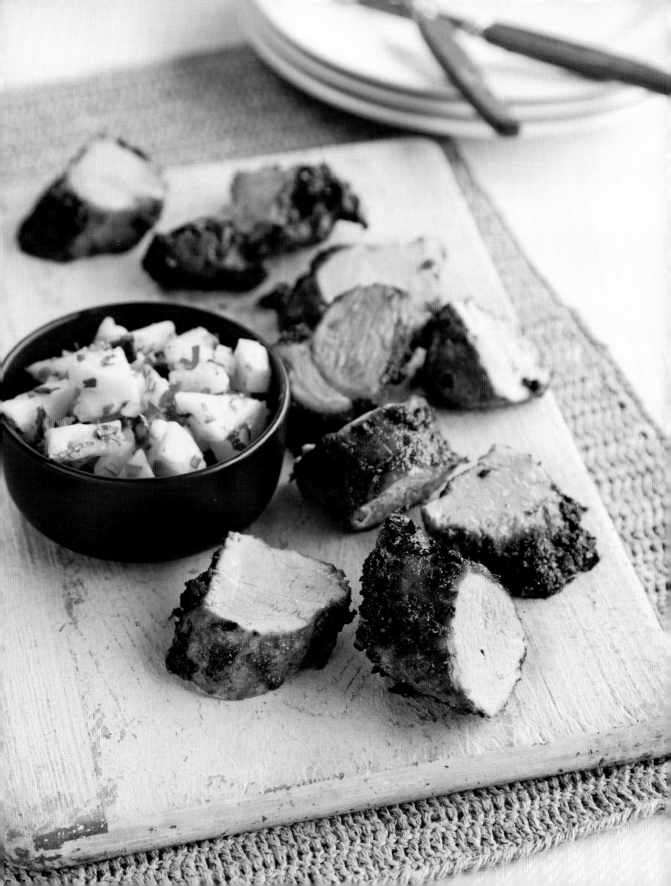

24 raw peeled large prawns,
deveined

FOR THE MARINADE

4 tablespoons garlic-infused
olive oil

2 teaspoons peeled and grated
fresh root ginger

1 bird's-eye chilli, deseeded
and sliced

4 kaffir lime leaves, torn

1 lemon grass stalk, finely
sliced

2 tablespoons Thai fish sauce

2 tablespoons lime juice

4 teaspoons soft light
brown sugar

salt and freshly ground
black pepper

TO GARNISH

1 tablespoon each chopped
fresh coriander, mint and
Thai basil leaves

1 large red chilli, deseeded
and sliced

PRAWNS WITH ASIAN DRESSING

**PREPARATION TIME: 10 MINUTES,
    PLUS MARINATING**
COOKING TIME: 6 MINUTES
SERVES: 4

Combine the marinade ingredients in a non-metallic dish. Add
the prawns and stir well, then leave to marinate for 30 minutes.
Meanwhile, soak 24 bamboo skewers in cold water for 30 minutes.

Thread 1 prawn on to each skewer and tip the marinade juices into
a small saucepan.

Cook the prawns on a hot barbecue or griddle pan for 2 minutes
on each side, then arrange on a platter.

Meanwhile, bring the marinade juices to a boil, then pour over
the prawns. Serve garnished with the herbs and chilli slices.

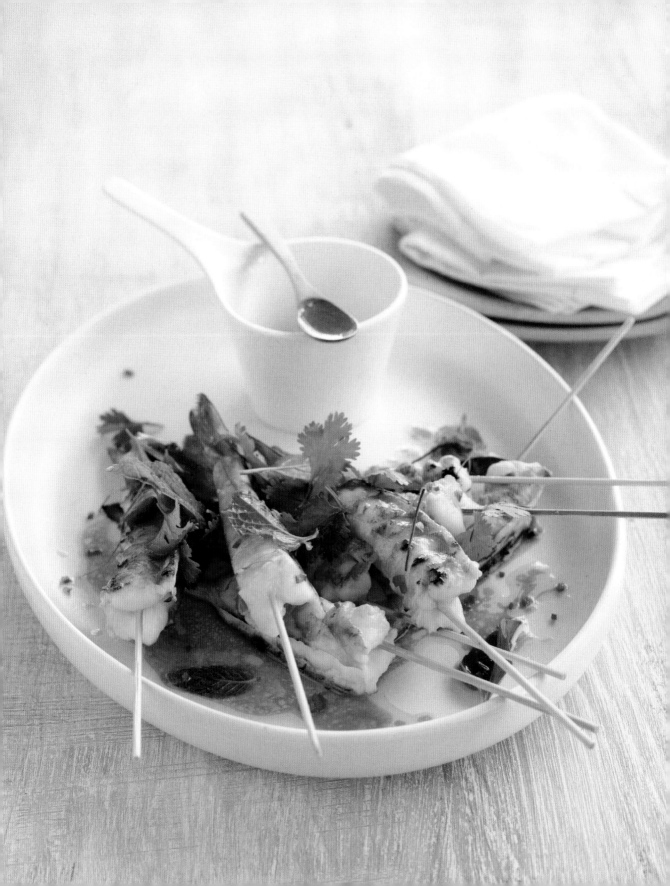

8 chicken drumsticks

2 tablespoons maple syrup

2 tablespoons olive oil

2 tablespoons dark soy sauce

1 teaspoon tomato purée

1 tablespoon Dijon mustard

chopped flat-leaf parsley,
to garnish

TO SERVE (OPTIONAL)

steamed rice

crisp green salad

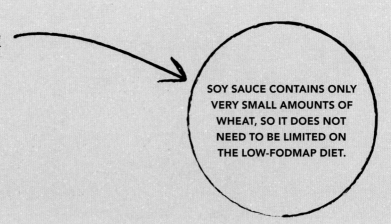

SOY SAUCE CONTAINS ONLY VERY SMALL AMOUNTS OF WHEAT, SO IT DOES NOT NEED TO BE LIMITED ON THE LOW-FODMAP DIET.

STICKY SOY-GLAZED DRUMSTICKS

PREPARATION TIME: 20 MINUTES
COOKING TIME: 30 MINUTES
SERVES: 4

Preheat the oven to 220°C (425°F), Gas Mark 7.

Put the drumsticks on to a board and make 4 deep slashes in each one along the thick part of the meat, cutting down to the bone on both sides.

Mix together the maple syrup, oil, soy sauce, tomato purée and mustard in a large bowl. Toss the drumsticks in the glaze, turning to coat the meat well.

Transfer the drumsticks to a roasting tin and roast at the top of the oven for 20–25 minutes or until the chicken is cooked through. Garnish with parsley and serve with steamed rice and a crisp green salad, if liked.

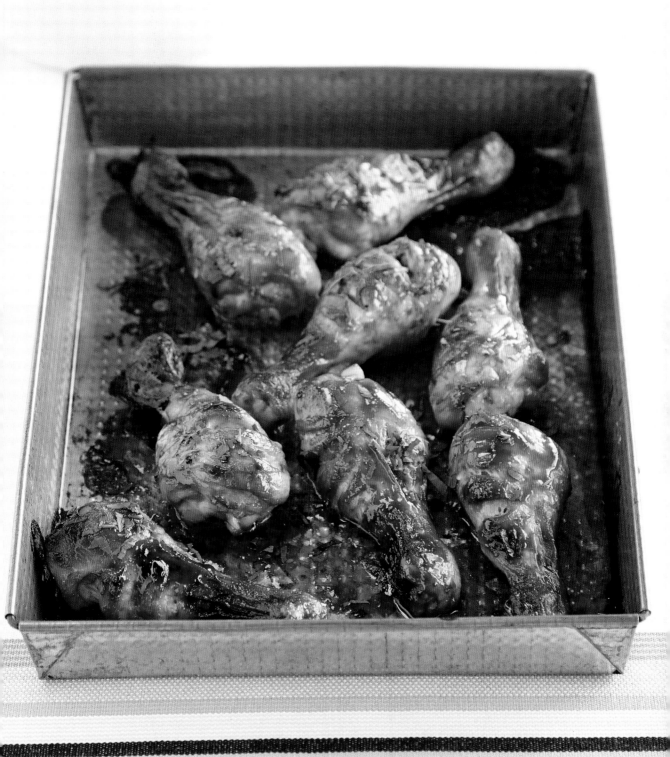

125ml (4fl oz) soy sauce

3 tablespoons smooth peanut butter (free from high-fructose corn syrup)

2 tablespoons water

2 chicken breasts, cut into strips

1 red pepper, deseeded and cut into chunks

1 yellow pepper, deseeded and cut into chunks

1 courgette, halved and sliced

½ Chinese cabbage, shredded

2 carrots, peeled and grated

25g (1oz) bean sprouts

small handful of fresh coriander leaves

2 teaspoons sesame oil

juice of 1 lime

2 tablespoons sesame seeds, toasted, to serve

CHICKEN & VEGETABLE SATAY

PREPARATION TIME: 20 MINUTES
COOKING TIME: 15 MINUTES
SERVES: 4

Preheat the grill on the highest setting. Soak 8 satay sticks in water.

Mix together the soy sauce, peanut butter and measured water in a large bowl. Add the chicken, peppers and courgette and toss them in the peanut butter mixture. Thread the chicken, peppers and courgette on to the soaked satay sticks.

Arrange the satay sticks on a baking sheet and grill for 12–14 minutes, turning regularly, until the chicken is cooked through.

Meanwhile, put the cabbage, grated carrot, bean sprouts and coriander leaves into a bowl with the sesame oil and lime juice and toss to coat.

Serve the satay with the salad, sprinkled with toasted sesame seeds.

6 thin slices of prosciutto

12 cleaned king scallops

4 long, thick sprigs
of rosemary

3 tablespoons olive oil

salt

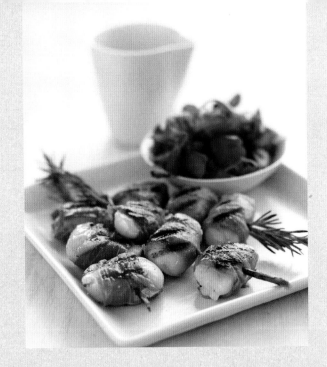

PROSCIUTTO, SCALLOP & ROSEMARY SKEWERS

PREPARATION TIME: 10 MINUTES
COOKING TIME: 5 MINUTES
SERVES: 4

Cut each slice of prosciutto in half lengthways. Wrap one piece around each scallop.

Strip the leaves from the bottom of each rosemary sprig, then thread 3 scallops on to each rosemary 'skewer'.

Drizzle over the oil and season with salt. Cook under a hot grill or on a hot barbecue for 5 minutes, or until just cooked through, turning once.

2 lemon grass stalks

1 tablespoon garlic-infused oil

4 tablespoons peeled and sliced fresh root ginger

1 red chilli

3 teaspoons soft light brown sugar

4 tablespoons Thai fish sauce

500g (1lb 2oz) beef steak strips

1 tablespoon oil

600g (1lb 5oz) fresh rice noodles

squeeze of lime juice

1/4 iceberg lettuce, shredded

2 carrots, grated

handful of mint leaves

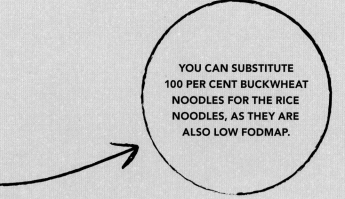

YOU CAN SUBSTITUTE 100 PER CENT BUCKWHEAT NOODLES FOR THE RICE NOODLES, AS THEY ARE ALSO LOW FODMAP.

GINGER BEEF SKEWERS

PREPARATION TIME: 15 MINUTES
COOKING TIME: 5 MINUTES
SERVES: 4

Put the lemon grass, garlic-infused oil, ginger, chilli, half the sugar and half the fish sauce into a blender and whizz to form a paste.

Rub the mixture all over the beef strips. Thread the meat on to skewers, then drizzle over the oil.

Heat a large griddle pan until smoking. Cook the skewered meat for 1–2 minutes on each side, until charred. Transfer to serving plates.

Meanwhile, cook the noodles according to the packet instructions. Cool the noodles under cold running water and drain.

Stir together the remaining sugar and fish sauce with the lime juice. Toss the mixture through the noodles along with the lettuce, carrots and mint leaves. Serve the mixture alongside the skewers.

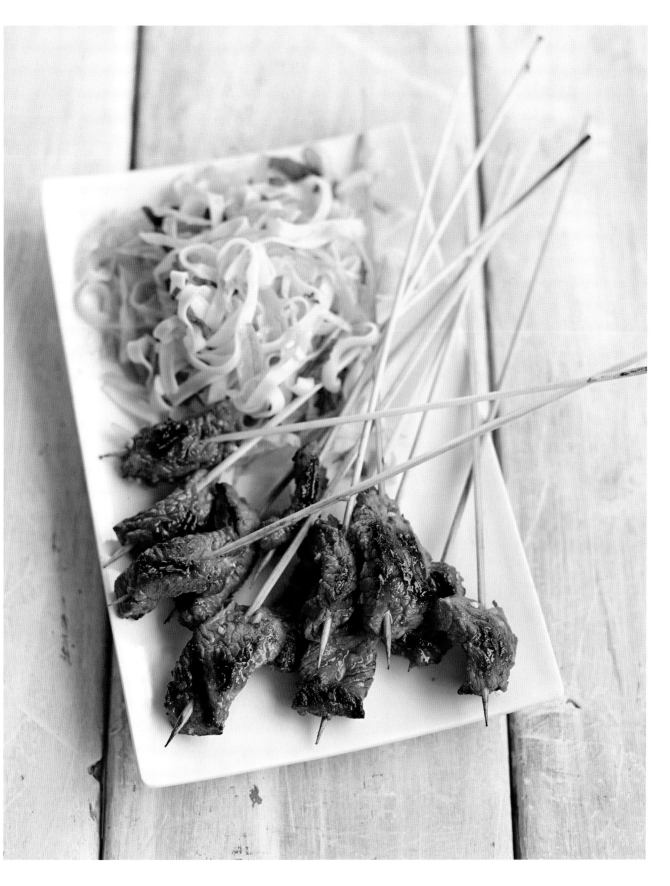

100g (3½oz) gluten-free plain flour

1 teaspoon gluten-free baking powder

½ teaspoon turmeric

2 teaspoons ground coriander

1 teaspoon ground cumin

1 teaspoon chilli powder

250ml (9fl oz) soda water, chilled

sunflower oil, for deep-frying

625g (1lb 6oz) courgettes, cut into thick batons

salt

plain lactose-free or plant-based yogurt (limit soya yogurt to 60g/2¼oz per portion), or standard yogurt if you know you tolerate lactose

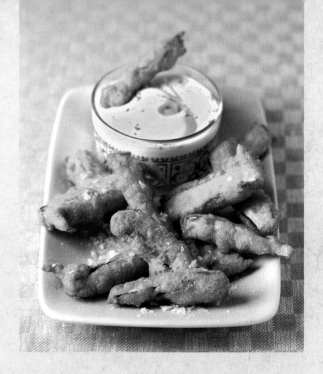

SPICED COURGETTE FRITTERS

PREPARATION TIME: 15 MINUTES
COOKING TIME: 10 MINUTES
SERVES: 4

Sift the flour, baking powder, turmeric, coriander, cumin and chilli powder into a large mixing bowl. Season with salt and gradually add the soda water to make a thick batter, being careful not to overmix.

Pour sunflower oil into a wok until it is one-third full and heat the oil to 180–190°C (350–375°F), or until a cube of bread immersed in the oil browns in 30 seconds.

Dip the courgette batons in the spiced batter, then deep-fry in batches for 1–2 minutes or until crisp and golden. Remove with a slotted spoon and drain on kitchen paper. Serve the courgettes immediately with the yogurt, to dip.

225g (8oz) firm tofu

1 tablespoon light soy sauce

1 tablespoon oyster sauce

1 tablespoon sesame oil

3 tablespoons chopped fresh coriander

1 small red chilli, deseeded and finely chopped

2.5cm (1 inch) piece of fresh root ginger, peeled and grated

2 teaspoons sesame seeds

125g (4½oz) bean sprouts

2 spring onions (green parts only), thinly sliced

1 tablespoon dark soy sauce

SILKEN TOFU IS HIGH IN FODMAPS AND SHOULD BE AVOIDED. FIRM TOFU IS FINE AS IT HAS A LOWER FODMAP CONTENT, BUT DISCARD THE WATER AS THIS IS THE PART THAT IS HIGHER IN FODMAPS.

ORIENTAL TOFU WITH SESAME SEEDS

PREPARATION TIME: 20 MINUTES, PLUS MARINATING
COOKING TIME: 5 MINUTES
SERVES: 4

Cut the tofu into 4 thin slices and put them into a bowl with the light soy sauce, oyster sauce, sesame oil, 2 tablespoons of the chopped coriander, the chilli and ginger and gently toss to mix. Cover the bowl with clingfilm and marinate in the refrigerator for 2 hours or overnight.

Remove the tofu from the marinade and place it on a plate. Scatter the sesame seeds over both sides of the tofu slices.

Heat a griddle pan until hot. Add the tofu and cook over medium heat for 1–2 minutes on each side, until scorched.

Toss the bean sprouts and spring onion with the dark soy sauce in a bowl, then divide the mixture between 4 small plates. Top with the hot tofu and sprinkle with the remaining chopped coriander. Serve as a starter.

MAIN
MEALS

pinch of saffron threads

1 tablespoon boiling water

4 skinless chicken drumsticks

4 skinless small chicken
thighs

1 lemon, halved

2 tablespoons maple syrup

150ml (¼ pint) dry white wine

125g (4½oz) green olives

salt and freshly ground black
pepper

2 tablespoons roughly chopped
flat-leaf parsley, to garnish

TO SERVE (OPTIONAL)

cooked new potatoes

cooked green beans (limit
each portion to 85g/3oz)

CHICKEN ROASTED
WITH LEMON, OLIVES & SAFFRON

PREPARATION TIME: 15 MINUTES
COOKING TIME: 25 MINUTES
SERVES: 4

Preheat the oven to 220°C (425°F), Gas Mark 7.

Soak the saffron threads in the measured boiling water in a small bowl.

Cut a couple of slashes across the top of each piece of chicken and
season with salt and pepper. Spread out the chicken in a large roasting
tin or ovenproof dish and squeeze over the lemon halves. Drizzle over
the maple syrup, pour over the saffron threads and soaking water
and add the white wine. Roast for 20 minutes, basting with the juices
occasionally. Add the olives and cook for a further 5 minutes, until the
chicken is cooked through.

Sprinkle with parsley and serve with new potatoes and green beans,
if liked.

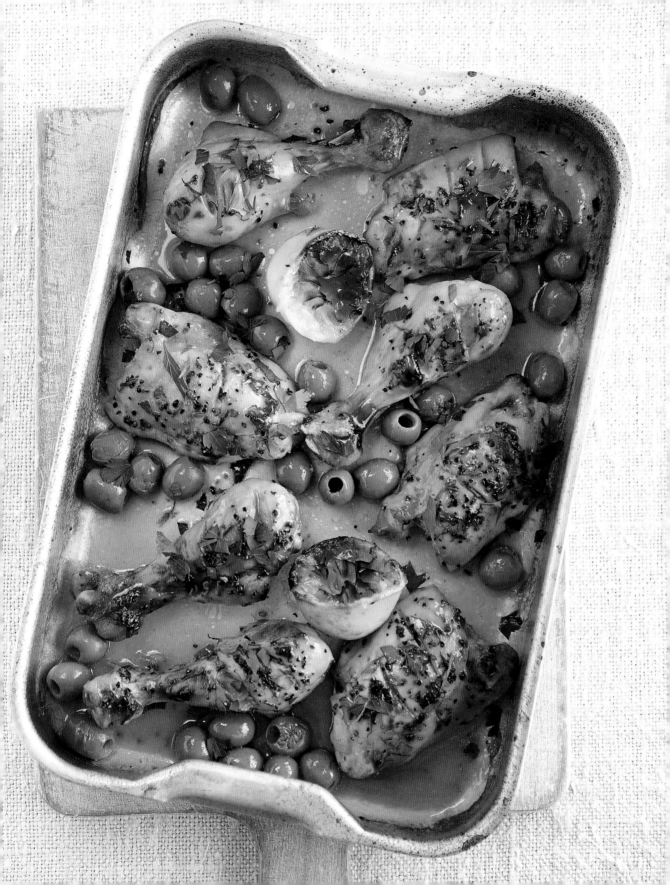

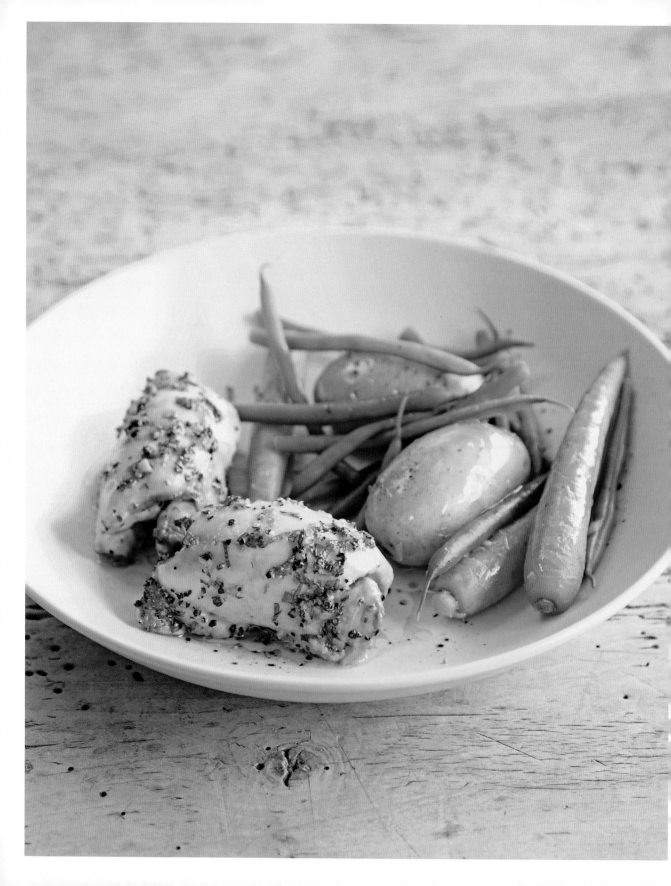

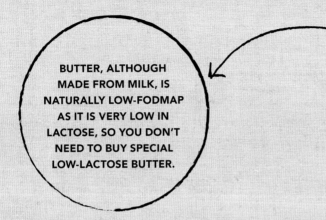

8 boneless, skinless chicken
thighs

finely grated zest and juice
of 1 lemon

3 tablespoons chopped
flat-leaf parsley

50g (1¾oz) butter

freshly ground black pepper

cooked seasonal vegetables,
to serve

BUTTER, ALTHOUGH
MADE FROM MILK, IS
NATURALLY LOW-FODMAP
AS IT IS VERY LOW IN
LACTOSE, SO YOU DON'T
NEED TO BUY SPECIAL
LOW-LACTOSE BUTTER.

BUTTER & LEMON ROASTED CHICKEN THIGHS

PREPARATION TIME: 10 MINUTES
COOKING TIME: 20–25 MINUTES
SERVES: 4

Preheat the oven to 200°C (400°F), Gas Mark 6.

Put the chicken thighs into a large bowl with the lemon zest and juice, parsley and plenty of pepper and mix well to coat the chicken. Roll each of the coated thighs back into shape and secure each with a cocktail stick.

Put the chicken thighs into a roasting tin, pouring any remaining juices over them, and top each with a small knob of butter. Roast for 20–25 minutes or until golden and cooked through. Serve with seasonal vegetables.

4 lamb loin chops, about 200g (7oz) each

1 tablespoon extra-virgin olive oil

4 teaspoons dried oregano

salt and freshly ground black pepper

rocket leaves, to garnish

FOR THE OLIVE & PINE NUT SALSA

3 tablespoons extra-virgin olive oil

25g (1oz) pine nuts, toasted

125g (4½oz) pitted black olives, halved

2 tablespoons drained capers in brine

2 tablespoons chopped flat-leaf parsley

1 tablespoon lemon juice

salt and freshly ground black pepper

LAMB
WITH OLIVE & PINE NUT SALSA

PREPARATION TIME: 10 MINUTES, PLUS COOLING

COOKING TIME: 10 MINUTES

SERVES: 4

Make the salsa. Heat 1 tablespoon of the oil in a small frying pan, add the pine nuts and cook gently for 30 seconds until golden. Leave to cool.

Combine the cooled pine nuts with the olives, capers, parsley, lemon juice and remaining oil in a bowl and season to taste with salt and pepper.

Heat a griddle pan until hot. Meanwhile, brush the chops with the oil and season with the oregano and salt and pepper. Transfer the chops to the hot griddle pan and cook over medium-high heat for 4 minutes on each side, until cooked.

Remove the chops from the pan, wrap loosely in kitchen foil and leave to rest for 5 minutes. Serve garnished with the rocket, with the salsa alongside.

4 aubergines

300g (10½oz) minced lamb

2 pinches of ground cinnamon

1 tablespoon garlic-infused olive oil

80g (2¾oz) cooked long-grain rice

20g (¾oz) pine nuts

1 bunch of spring onions (green parts only), chopped

2 tablespoons finely chopped mint

2 tablespoons finely chopped flat-leaf parsley

salt and freshly ground black pepper

> GARLIC-INFUSED OLIVE OIL IS LOW FODMAP AS THE FRUCTANS IN GARLIC ARE WATER-SOLUBLE AND THEREFORE DO NOT ENTER INTO THE OIL, SO YOU GET ALL THE GARLIC TASTE WITH NONE OF THE FODMAPS.

AUBERGINES STUFFED
WITH LAMB

PREPARATION TIME: 15 MINUTES
COOKING TIME: 35 MINUTES
SERVES: 4

Preheat the oven to 180°C (350°F), Gas Mark 4.

Rinse and dry the aubergines, then halve them lengthways and hollow out some of the flesh with a small spoon. Place the hollowed-out aubergines on a baking tray and bake for around 10 minutes, until slightly softened.

Season the minced lamb with the cinnamon and salt and pepper to taste.

Heat the oil in a nonstick saucepan. Add the lamb, rice, pine nuts, spring onion, chopped mint and parsley and mix well. Cook for 8–10 minutes, until the lamb is browned and the liquid has evaporated.

Fill the recesses in the aubergines with this mixture. Return the aubergines to the oven and bake for around 15 minutes, until piping hot. If necessary, add a little water in the bottom of the dish to ensure they do not stick. Serve warm or cold.

AUBERGINE & HARISSA SAUTÉ

PREPARATION TIME: 15 MINUTES
COOKING TIME: 10 MINUTES
SERVES: 4

4 tablespoons sunflower oil

750g (1lb 10oz) baby aubergines, thinly sliced

4 tomatoes, chopped

1 teaspoon ground cinnamon

1 teaspoon finely chopped fresh coriander leaves

2 tablespoons Low-FODMAP Harissa Paste (see below)

salt and freshly ground black pepper

cooked basmati rice, to serve

Heat the oil in a large frying pan and add the aubergines. Fry over high heat for 2–3 minutes, then add the tomatoes, cinnamon, coriander and harissa. Stir-fry for 3–4 minutes or until the aubergines are tender.

Season to taste and serve with basmati rice.

LOW-FODMAP HARISSA PASTE

Shop-bought harissa paste contains garlic and is off-limits for those following the low-FODMAP diet. This homemade alternative is delicious and easy to make.

In advance of making the paste, soak 8–10 dried red chillies in water for 2 days. To make the paste, dry-fry 2 teaspoons each of cumin and coriander seeds in a heavy-based frying pan over medium heat for 2–3 minutes, until they release a nutty aroma, then grind them to a powder using a pestle and mortar. Drain the chillies, chop off the stems, and squeeze out most of the seeds. Discard the stems and seeds and coarsely chop the chillies. Pound the chillies with 1–2 teaspoons of sea salt using a pestle and mortar. Add the ground spices and pound again, then beat in 3 tablespoons of garlic-infused olive oil. Spoon the paste into a sterilized jar and pour over another tablespoon of the oil. Seal and store in a cool place or in the refrigerator. Use within 2 months.

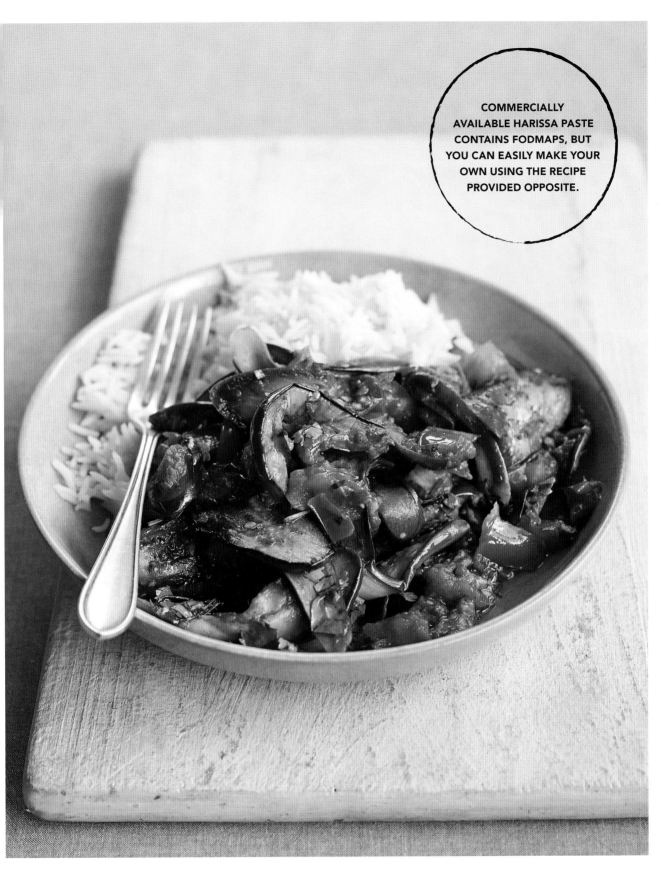

COMMERCIALLY AVAILABLE HARISSA PASTE CONTAINS FODMAPS, BUT YOU CAN EASILY MAKE YOUR OWN USING THE RECIPE PROVIDED OPPOSITE.

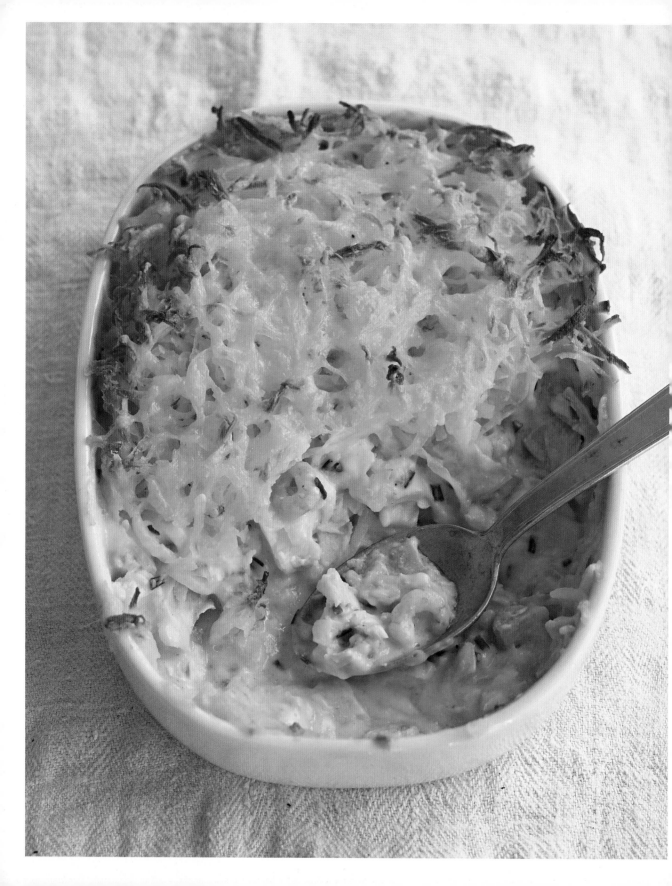

750g (1lb 10oz) potatoes, unpeeled

250g (9oz) white fish fillet (such as coley, pollack or haddock), cut into bite-sized pieces

250g (9oz) salmon fillet, cut into bite-sized pieces

400ml (14fl oz) hot lactose-free or plant-based milk (limit soya to 60ml/ 4 tablespoons per portion), or standard milk if you know you tolerate lactose

50g (1¾oz) butter

50g (1¾oz) gluten-free flour

100g (3½oz) Cheddar cheese, grated

2 teaspoons lemon juice

2 tablespoons chopped chives

100g (3½oz) small cooked peeled prawns (optional)

salt and freshly ground black pepper

EASY FISH PIE
WITH CRUNCHY POTATO TOPPING

PREPARATION TIME: 20 MINUTES
COOKING TIME: 30 MINUTES
SERVES: 4

Preheat the oven to 180°C (350°F), Gas Mark 4.

Cook the potatoes in a large saucepan of lightly salted water for 6–7 minutes. Drain and set aside to cool slightly.

Meanwhile, place the white fish and salmon in a deep-sided frying pan. Pour over the hot milk and bring to a boil. Reduce the heat and simmer gently for 3–4 minutes, until the fish is just cooked. Strain the milk into a jug and transfer the fish to an ovenproof dish.

Put the butter and flour into a saucepan and warm gently to melt the butter. Stir for 2 minutes to cook the flour.

Add the reserved milk to the saucepan a little at a time, stirring well to incorporate it. Stir for a further 2–3 minutes, until thickened, then remove from the heat and stir in half the cheese, the lemon juice and the chives, and season to taste. Pour the sauce over the fish, add the prawns, if using, and stir gently to coat.

Wearing rubber gloves to protect your hands from the heat, grate the potatoes coarsely and scatter the grated potato over the fish. Sprinkle over the remaining cheese and bake for 15–20 minutes, until the topping is golden and crispy.

3 tablespoons gluten-free
plain flour
....
1 large egg, beaten
....
30g (1oz) gluten-free
breadcrumbs
....
25g (1oz) polenta
....
500g (1lb 2oz) cod fillet, cut
into 8 thick pieces
....
3 tablespoons sunflower oil

GLUTEN-FREE FLOURS AND BREADCRUMBS ARE RECOMMENDED BECAUSE GLUTEN-FREE PRODUCTS ARE GENERALLY WHEAT-FREE AND THEREFORE LOW FODMAP.

HOMEMADE FISH FINGERS

PREPARATION TIME: 10 MINUTES
COOKING TIME: 10 MINUTES
SERVES: 4

Put the flour and the beaten egg into 2 separate shallow bowls, then mix the breadcrumbs and polenta together in a third bowl.

Gently toss the pieces of fish first in the flour, then in the egg and finally in the breadcrumb and polenta mixture to coat.

Heat the sunflower oil in a frying pan over medium heat. Add the fish fingers carefully and cook for 5–6 minutes, turning occasionally, until golden. Drain on kitchen paper before serving.

625g (1lb 6oz) skinless haddock fillet

600ml (20fl oz) lactose-free or plant-based milk (limit soya to 60ml/4 tablespoons per portion), or standard milk if you know you tolerate lactose

1 bay leaf

40g (1½oz) butter

40g (1½oz) gluten-free plain flour

50g (1¾oz) Gruyère cheese, grated

½ teaspoon English mustard

salad, to serve

FOR THE TOPPING

100g (3½oz) fresh gluten-free breadcrumbs

25g (1oz) Gruyère cheese, finely grated

finely grated zest of 1 lemon

2 tablespoons chopped flat-leaf parsley

CREAMY HADDOCK GRATIN

PREPARATION TIME: 10 MINUTES
COOKING TIME: 25 MINUTES
SERVES: 4

Preheat the oven to 220°C (425°F), Gas Mark 7.

Place the haddock in a saucepan with the milk and bay leaf, bring to a boil, then boil for 3 minutes. Remove the fish with a slotted spoon, reserving the milk, and divide it between 4 individual gratin dishes.

Melt the butter in a separate saucepan, then add the flour and cook over medium heat, stirring, for a few seconds. Remove from the heat and add the reserved milk, a little at a time, stirring well between each addition. Return the pan to the heat, bring to a boil and cook, stirring constantly, until thickened. Remove the pan from the heat and mix in the grated Gruyère and mustard.

Pour the sauce over the fish, dividing it evenly between the dishes. Mix together the ingredients for the topping and scatter over the sauce. Place on the top shelf of the oven and bake for 10 minutes, until the topping is golden and the sauce is bubbling. Serve with a simple salad.

1 mild green chilli, deseeded and chopped

1 teaspoon ground coriander

½ teaspoon turmeric

2.5cm (1 inch) piece of fresh root ginger, peeled and sliced

1 teaspoon garlic-infused oil

1 tablespoon coconut oil

1 bunch of spring onions (green parts only), sliced

1 teaspoon cumin seeds

150ml (¼ pint) coconut milk

250ml (9fl oz) water

450g (1lb) mackerel fillets, cut into 5cm (2 inch) pieces

small handful of fresh coriander leaves, roughly torn

salt and freshly ground black pepper

cooked basmati rice, to serve (optional)

MACKEREL CURRY

PREPARATION TIME: 15 MINUTES
COOKING TIME: 20 MINUTES
SERVES: 4

Place the chilli, ground coriander, turmeric, ginger and garlic-infused oil in a small blender and blend together to a smooth paste.

Heat the coconut oil in a wok or large frying pan over medium heat. Add the spice paste, spring onions and cumin seeds and cook for 2–3 minutes, until the spices are fragrant.

Pour in the coconut milk and measured water. Bring to a boil, then simmer for 5 minutes. Season with salt and pepper.

Add the mackerel pieces to the wok or frying pan and cook for 6–8 minutes, until the fish is cooked, then stir in the coriander leaves. Serve immediately, with basmati rice, if liked.

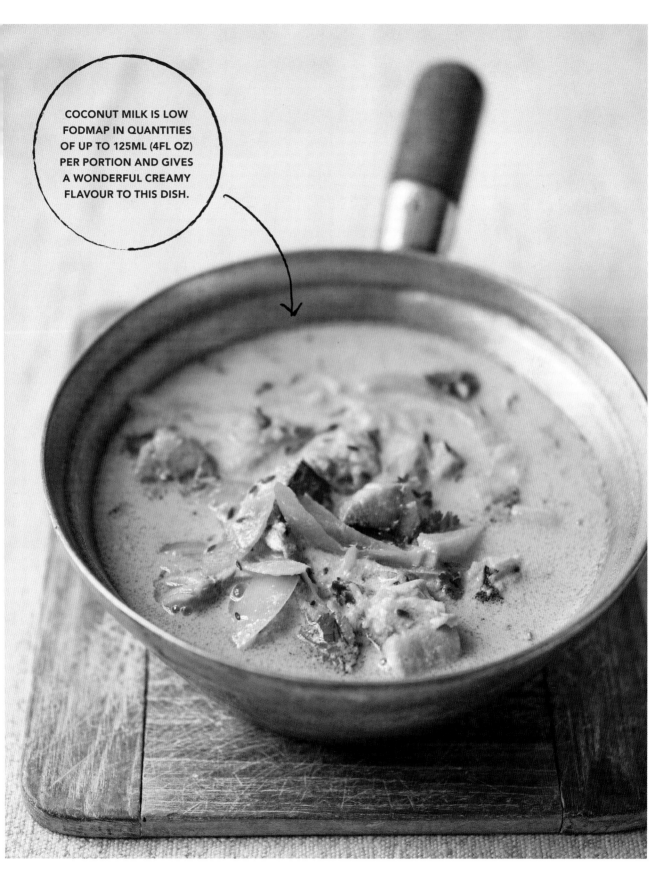

COCONUT MILK IS LOW FODMAP IN QUANTITIES OF UP TO 125ML (4FL OZ) PER PORTION AND GIVES A WONDERFUL CREAMY FLAVOUR TO THIS DISH.

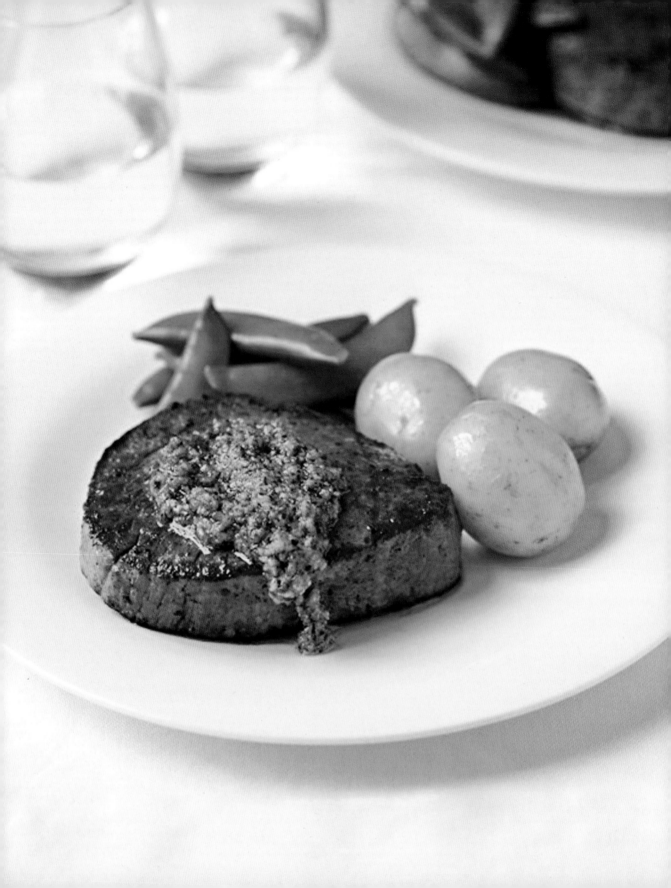

2 pieces of beef fillet, about 200g (7oz) each

salt and freshly ground black pepper

steamed new potatoes, to serve

FOR THE PESTO

50g (1¾oz) toasted walnuts

3 tablespoons chopped mixed herbs (such as coriander, parsley and basil)

2 tablespoons grated Parmesan cheese

2 tablespoons garlic-infused olive oil

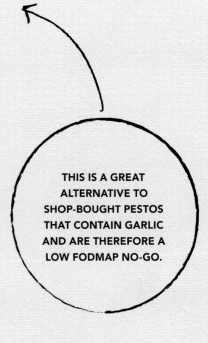

THIS IS A GREAT ALTERNATIVE TO SHOP-BOUGHT PESTOS THAT CONTAIN GARLIC AND ARE THEREFORE A LOW FODMAP NO-GO.

BEEF FILLET
WITH WALNUT PESTO

PREPARATION TIME: 20 MINUTES
COOKING TIME: 5 MINUTES
SERVES: 2

Heat a griddle pan or a heavy-based frying pan. Season the meat with salt and pepper, add it to the pan and cook over high heat for 2 minutes on each side or until cooked to your liking.

Meanwhile, make the pesto. Put all the ingredients into the bowl of a food processor or blender and process until combined but still textured.

Serve the cooked steaks with the sauce spooned on top, with steamed new potatoes alongside.

HORSERADISH BEEF
WITH QUINOA

PREPARATION TIME: 15 MINUTES, PLUS RESTING
COOKING TIME: 20 MINUTES
SERVES: 4

625g (1lb 6oz) beef fillet, rolled and tied

1 tablespoon horseradish sauce

2 tablespoons olive oil

300g (10½oz) quinoa

1 green pepper, deseeded and sliced

1 bunch of spring onions (green parts only), thinly sliced

1 tablespoon chopped flat-leaf parsley

1 tablespoon chopped mint

40g (1½oz) rocket

Preheat the oven to 200°C (400° F), Gas Mark 6.

Brush the beef with the horseradish sauce.

Heat 1 tablespoon of the oil in a frying pan over high heat. Add the beef and sear on all sides, until browned. Transfer the beef to a roasting tin and bake for 20 minutes, until cooked to your liking. Cover the tin with kitchen foil and leave to rest for 5–6 minutes, then slice the beef.

Meanwhile, cook the quinoa in a saucepan of boiling water for 8–9 minutes, or according to the packet instructions.

Heat the remaining oil in a large frying pan. Add the pepper and cook for 3–4 minutes over medium heat until softened, then add the spring onion and cook for a further minute. Remove the pan from the heat and stir in the chopped herbs.

Drain the quinoa and stir it into the peppers, spring onion and herbs mixture. Divide the mixture between 4 warmed plates and top with the rocket and sliced beef.

500g (1lb 2oz) minced pork

2 spring onions (green parts only), finely chopped, plus extra to garnish

1 tablespoon peeled and very finely chopped fresh root ginger

1 tablespoon cornflour

1 small egg white, whisked

3–4 tablespoons vegetable or groundnut oil

350g (12oz) jasmine rice

salt

soy sauce, to serve (optional)

FOR THE SWEET & SOUR SAUCE

225g (8oz) can pineapple chunks in juice

125g (4½oz) tomato ketchup (free from fructose, onion and garlic)

2½ tablespoons soft light brown sugar

2 tablespoons malt vinegar

2 teaspoons light soy sauce

MINCED PORK BALLS
WITH SWEET & SOUR SAUCE

PREPARATION TIME: 15 MINUTES
COOKING TIME: 30–40 MINUTES
SERVES: 4

Put the minced pork into a large bowl with the spring onions and ginger. Whisk the cornflour into the egg white and add the mixture to the pork, mixing until well combined. Form the mixture into 20–24 balls.

Heat the oil in a large nonstick frying pan. Cook the meatballs over medium-high heat for 10–12 minutes, until cooked through and golden.

Meanwhile, place the rice in a saucepan with 1½ times its volume of cold water. Bring to a boil, season with salt, cover the pan with a lid and simmer gently for 11–14 minutes, until the rice is tender and the liquid has been absorbed. Garnish with spring onion.

Make the sweet and sour sauce. Tip the pineapple and its juice into a mini-chopper or food processor and pulse until crushed but not smooth. (Alternatively, chop it finely by hand.) Pour the crushed pineapple into a small pan with the remaining ingredients and bring the mixture to a boil, then reduce the heat and simmer gently for 5–7 minutes, until thickened.

Drain the excess oil from the pan of meatballs, then pour the sauce into the pan and simmer for 1–2 minutes, until the meatballs are well coated in the sauce. Spoon the meatballs and sauce over the rice and serve immediately with soy sauce, if desired.

2 tablespoons maple syrup

2 tablespoons dark soy sauce

2 teaspoons Chinese five-spice powder

1 teaspoon Szechuan pepper, lightly crushed

1 teaspoon peeled and finely grated fresh root ginger

2 teaspoons sesame oil

500g (1lb 2oz) pork tenderloin, thickly sliced

1 red pepper, deseeded and thinly sliced

350g (12oz) Chinese cabbage, thinly sliced

200g (7oz) bean sprouts

350g (12oz) baby pak choi, halved lengthways

2 teaspoons sesame seeds, to serve

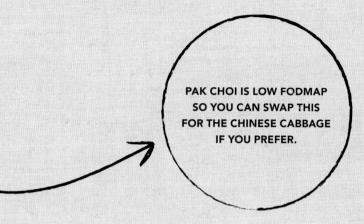

PAK CHOI IS LOW FODMAP SO YOU CAN SWAP THIS FOR THE CHINESE CABBAGE IF YOU PREFER.

CHINESE PORK & VEGETABLES

PREPARATION TIME: 15 MINUTES
COOKING TIME: 20 MINUTES
SERVES: 4

Mix together the maple syrup, soy sauce, Chinese five-spice powder, Szechuan pepper, ginger and 1 teaspoon of the sesame oil in a bowl. Add the pork to the bowl and massage the meat well with the mixture.

Heat a large, nonstick frying pan over medium-high heat, then scrape the pork mixture into the pan and cook for 4–5 minutes, turning occasionally, until the pork is just cooked and tender.

Meanwhile, heat the remaining sesame oil in a wok over medium-high heat, then add the red pepper, Chinese cabbage, bean sprouts and baby pak choi and stir-fry for 2–3 minutes, until just tender.

Remove the pork from the heat and serve immediately, sprinkled with the sesame seeds, with the stir-fried vegetables alongside.

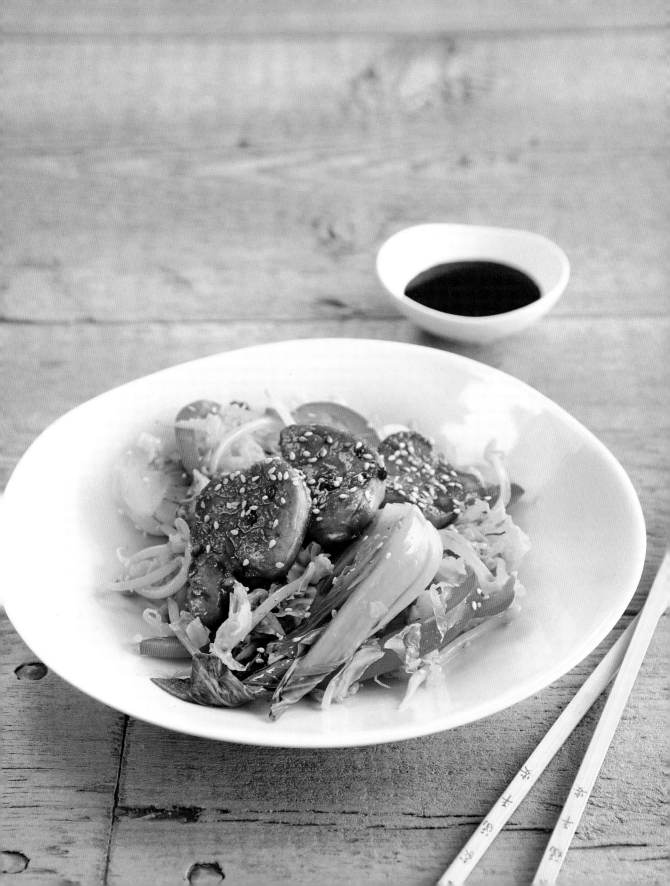

1 tablespoon garlic-infused oil

1 bunch of spring onions (green parts only), sliced

1–2 hot green chillies, deseeded and sliced

5–6 fresh curry leaves

1 tablespoon mild Low-FODMAP Curry Powder (see page 47)

¼ teaspoon turmeric

½ teaspoon fenugreek seeds

4 carrots, peeled and cut into thin matchsticks

250g (9oz) green beans, trimmed and halved

400ml (14fl oz) can coconut milk

juice of 1 lime

salt and freshly ground black pepper

steamed rice or gluten-free bread, to serve (optional)

UNLIKE OTHER BEANS, GREEN BEANS ARE LOW FODMAP IF EATEN IN MODERATE PORTIONS OF 85G (3OZ) OR LESS.

SPICED CARROT & GREEN BEAN STEW

PREPARATION TIME: 10 MINUTES
COOKING TIME: 20 MINUTES
SERVES: 4

Heat the oil in a heavy-based saucepan. Add the spring onions, chillies and curry leaves and cook over medium heat for 1–2 minutes, until fragrant. Sprinkle over the curry powder, turmeric and fenugreek seeds and season well.

Add the carrots and beans and cook, stirring, for a further 3–4 minutes, until everything is coated in the spices. Reduce the heat to low, pour over the coconut milk and simmer for 10–12 minutes or until the vegetables are tender.

Remove the saucepan from the heat and stir in the lime juice. Ladle the stew into warm bowls and serve with steamed rice or gluten-free bread, if liked.

butter or oil, for greasing

625g (1lb 6oz) potatoes,
thinly sliced

500g (1lb 2oz) spinach leaves

200g (7oz) mozzarella cheese,
grated

4 vine tomatoes, sliced

3 eggs, beaten

300ml (½ pint) whipping cream

salt and freshly ground black
pepper

crisp salad, to serve

SPINACH & POTATO GRATIN

PREPARATION TIME: 10 MINUTES
COOKING TIME: 35 MINUTES
SERVES: 4

Preheat the oven to 180°C (350°F), Gas Mark 4. Grease a large ovenproof dish.

Cook the potato slices in a large saucepan of salted boiling water for 5 minutes, then drain well.

Meanwhile, cook the spinach in a separate saucepan of boiling water for 1–2 minutes. Drain and squeeze out the excess water.

Arrange half the potato slices in a layer in the prepared ovenproof dish. Cover this layer with the spinach and half the mozzarella, seasoning each layer well with salt and pepper. Cover with the remaining potato slices and arrange the tomato slices on top. Sprinkle with the remaining mozzarella.

Whisk the eggs and cream together in a bowl and season well with salt and pepper. Pour this mixture over the ingredients in the dish. Bake for about 30 minutes. Serve immediately with a salad.

4 tablespoons vegetable oil

1 bunch of spring onions
(green parts only), thinly
sliced

1 red chilli, slit lengthways
and deseeded

3cm (1½ inch) piece of
fresh root ginger, peeled
and shredded

2 plum tomatoes, finely chopped

1 tablespoon Low-FODMAP Curry
Powder (see page 47)

200ml (7fl oz) canned coconut
milk

800g (1lb 12oz) fresh clams,
scrubbed

1 large handful of chopped
coriander leaves

3 tablespoons grated fresh
coconut

TO SERVE (OPTIONAL)

salad

gluten-free crusty bread

COCONUT SPICED CLAMS

PREPARATION TIME: 15 MINUTES
COOKING TIME: 20 MINUTES
SERVES: 4

Heat the oil in a large wok or saucepan until hot. Add the spring onions, red chilli and ginger and stir-fry over medium heat for 3–4 minutes. Increase the heat to high, stir in the tomatoes, curry powder and coconut milk and cook for a further 4–5 minutes.

Add the clams to the pan, discarding any that have cracked or don't shut when tapped, stir to mix and cover the pan tightly with a lid, then continue to cook over high heat for 6–8 minutes, until the clams have opened. Discard any that remain closed.

Stir the chopped coriander into the saucepan and sprinkle over the grated coconut. Ladle the mixture into bowls and serve immediately, with a fresh salad and crusty bread to mop up the juices, if liked.

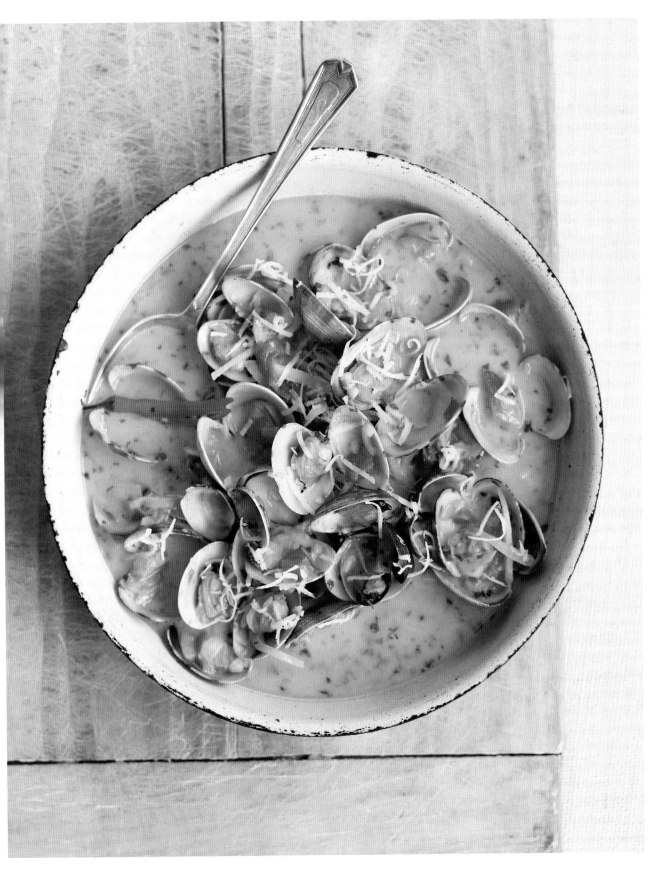

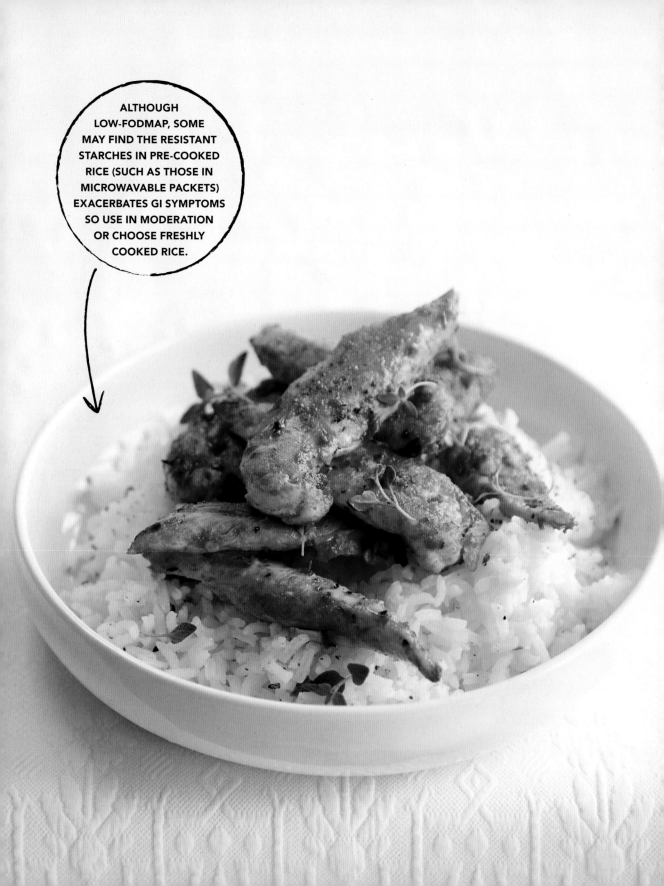

ALTHOUGH LOW-FODMAP, SOME MAY FIND THE RESISTANT STARCHES IN PRE-COOKED RICE (SUCH AS THOSE IN MICROWAVABLE PACKETS) EXACERBATES GI SYMPTOMS SO USE IN MODERATION OR CHOOSE FRESHLY COOKED RICE.

2 tablespoons olive oil

500g (1lb 2oz) small chicken fillets

sprigs of thyme, to garnish

FOR THE PIRI-PIRI SAUCE

1 teaspoon very finely chopped red chilli

1 tablespoon garlic-infused olive oil

$\frac{1}{4}$ teaspoon dried oregano

$\frac{1}{4}$ teaspoon dried thyme

1 teaspoon paprika

2 tablespoons red wine vinegar

TO SERVE

steamed rice

crisp green salad (optional)

PIRI PIRI STIR-FRY

PREPARATION TIME: 5 MINUTES
COOKING TIME: 10 MINUTES
SERVES: 4

Heat the oil in a large, heavy-based wok or frying pan. Add the chicken and cook over high heat, stirring occasionally, for 5 minutes or until golden in places.

Mix together the piri-piri sauce ingredients in a bowl and pour the mixture into the pan with the chicken. Stir-fry for a further 3–4 minutes, stirring occasionally, until the sauce flavours the chicken and the chicken is cooked through. Garnish with fresh thyme sprigs.

Serve hot with steamed rice and a crisp green salad, if liked.

3 tablespoons light soy sauce

1 tablespoon peeled and finely grated fresh root ginger

500g (1lb 2oz) firm tofu, cut into 15mm (⅝inch) slices

2 tablespoons vegetable or groundnut oil

1 carrot, peeled and cut into fine matchsticks

500g (1lb 2oz) pak choi, sliced

200g (7oz) bean sprouts

225g (8oz) can bamboo shoots in water

4 tablespoons oyster sauce

2 teaspoons golden sesame seeds, to garnish (optional)

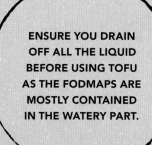

ENSURE YOU DRAIN OFF ALL THE LIQUID BEFORE USING TOFU AS THE FODMAPS ARE MOSTLY CONTAINED IN THE WATERY PART.

MARINATED TOFU
WITH VEGETABLES

PREPARATION TIME: 15 MINUTES, PLUS MARINATING
COOKING TIME: 15 MINUTES
SERVES: 4

Mix the soy sauce and ginger in a small bowl. Arrange the tofu slices in a shallow dish and pour over the marinade, turning to coat. Set aside to marinate for about 20 minutes.

Preheat the grill on the highest setting. Line a grill rack with kitchen foil.

Carefully transfer the tofu slices to the foil-lined grill rack, reserving the marinade. Cook under the hot grill for about 3 minutes on each side, until golden. Remove from the heat and keep warm.

Meanwhile, heat the oil in a wok over medium heat. Add the carrot and pak choi and stir-fry for 4–5 minutes, until beginning to soften. Add the bean sprouts and bamboo shoots and cook for 1 minute, then pour in the remaining marinade and the oyster sauce.

Spoon the vegetables into deep bowls, top with the grilled tofu slices and sprinkle with golden sesame seeds, if using. Serve immediately.

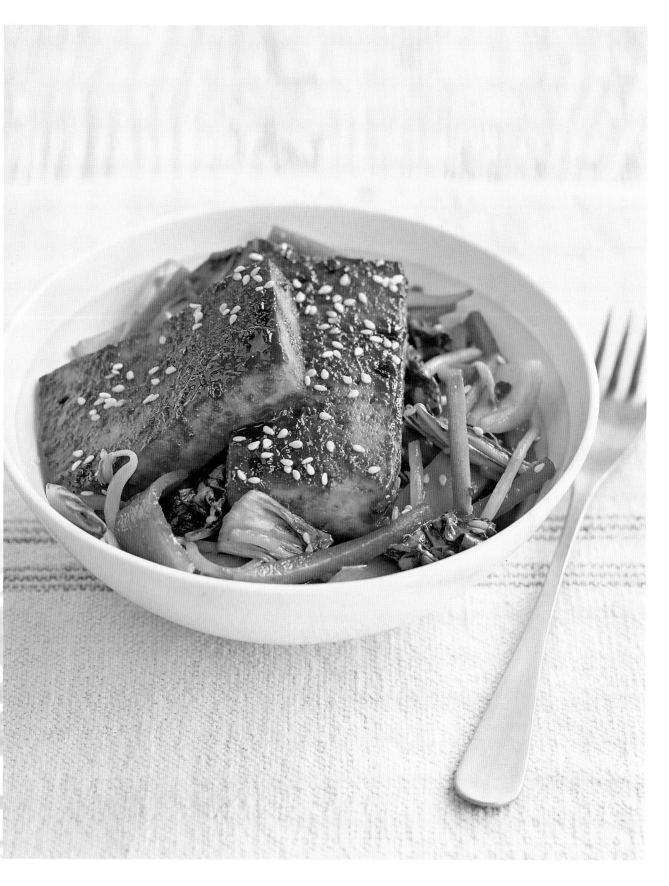

300g (10½oz) gluten-free penne

5½ tablespoons olive oil

75g (2¾oz) Parmesan cheese, grated

handful of tarragon leaves

55g (2oz) pine nuts, toasted

grated zest and juice of 1 lemon

3 tablespoons garlic-infused olive oil

3 cooked chicken breasts, sliced

100g (3½oz) watercress

12 baby tomatoes, quartered

CHICKEN & TARRAGON PESTO PENNE

PREPARATION TIME: 20 MINUTES
COOKING TIME: 10 MINUTES
SERVES: 4

Cook the penne in a large saucepan of boiling water for 8–9 minutes or according to the packet instructions. Drain and refresh under cold running water, then toss with 2 tablespoons of the olive oil.

Meanwhile, put the Parmesan, tarragon, pine nuts and lemon zest into the bowl of a food processor and blend for 1 minute. Then, with the motor running, gradually pour in the remaining olive oil and the garlic-infused olive oil to form the pesto.

Transfer the pasta to a serving bowl. Add the chicken, watercress, tomatoes, lemon juice and pesto and toss to mix. Serve immediately.

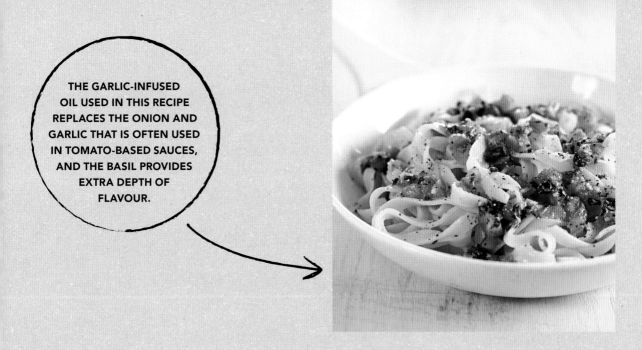

THE GARLIC-INFUSED OIL USED IN THIS RECIPE REPLACES THE ONION AND GARLIC THAT IS OFTEN USED IN TOMATO-BASED SAUCES, AND THE BASIL PROVIDES EXTRA DEPTH OF FLAVOUR.

PASTA
WITH TOMATO & BASIL SAUCE

PREPARATION TIME: 5 MINUTES
COOKING TIME: 10 MINUTES
SERVES: 4

400g (14oz) gluten-free spaghetti

3 tablespoons garlic-infused olive oil

2 tablespoons olive oil

6 ripe vine tomatoes, deseeded and chopped

25g (1oz) basil leaves

salt and freshly ground black pepper

Cook the pasta in a large saucepan of salted boiling water according to the packet instructions.

Drain the pasta and return it to the pan. Add the oils, chopped tomatoes and basil leaves. Season to taste with salt and pepper and toss well to mix. Serve immediately.

375g (13oz) gluten-free fusilli

50g (1¾oz) pine nuts, toasted,
1 tablespoon reserved to
garnish

150g (5½oz) watercress, plus
extra sprigs to serve

5 tablespoons extra-virgin
olive oil

2 tablespoons garlic-infused
olive oil

150g (5½oz) crumbly
low-lactose goats' cheese,
plus extra to serve

salt and freshly ground black
pepper

SOME VARIETIES OF GOATS' CHEESE ARE HIGHER IN LACTOSE THAN OTHERS. CHECK THE LABEL AND OPT FOR THOSE THAT CONTAIN LESS THAN 1 GRAM OF LACTOSE (LABELLED AS SUGAR) PER 100 GRAMS OF CHEESE.

GOATS' CHEESE & WATERCRESS PESTO PASTA

PREPARATION TIME: 10 MINUTES
COOKING TIME: 10–12 MINUTES
SERVES: 4

Cook the pasta in a large saucepan of salted boiling water according to the packet instructions, until al dente.

Meanwhile, put the pine nuts and watercress into the bowl of a food processor with a generous pinch of salt. Process for 15 seconds until roughly chopped. Then, with the motor running, drizzle in the oils while you process for a further 20 seconds.

Drain the pasta thoroughly and tip it into a bowl. Crumble in the goats' cheese and stir well. Season with pepper, then stir the pesto into the hot pasta. Divide the pasta between 4 serving plates and serve immediately with the reserved goats' cheese, pine nuts and some watercress sprigs.

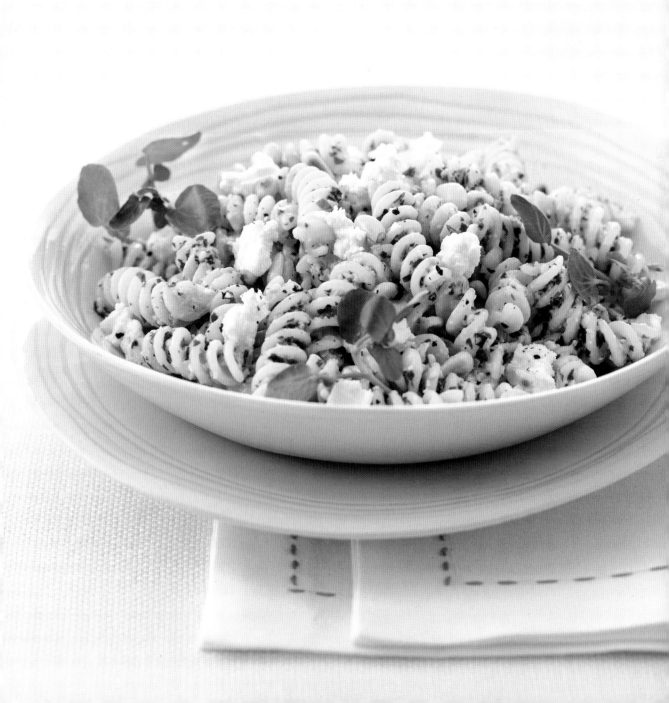

2 tablespoons garlic-infused
olive oil

....

1 bunch of spring onions
(green parts only), chopped

....

400g (14oz) can cherry
tomatoes

....

½ teaspoon chilli flakes

....

pinch of sugar

....

½ teaspoon finely grated
lemon zest

....

350g (12oz) gluten-free
linguine or spaghetti

....

2 x 120g (4¼oz) cans
sardines in oil, drained

....

2 teaspoons rinsed capers

....

salt and freshly ground
black pepper

....

basil leaves, to garnish
(optional)

SPICY SARDINE LINGUINE

PREPARATION TIME: 5 MINUTES
COOKING TIME: 20 MINUTES
SERVES: 4

Heat the olive oil in a large saucepan. Add the spring onions and cook over medium heat for 1 minute, until softened. Add the tomatoes, chilli flakes, sugar and lemon zest and season with salt and pepper. Bring to a boil, then cover the pan with a lid and simmer for about 10 minutes, until thickened. Stir the sardines and capers into the tomato sauce for the final 1–2 minutes of the cooking time.

Meanwhile, cook the linguine in a large saucepan of boiling salted water according to the packet instructions, until al dente. Drain, reserving 2 tablespoons of the cooking water, and return the pasta to the pan.

When the tomato sauce is ready, add it to the drained pasta along with the reserved cooking water and toss gently. Serve the mixture heaped in bowls, garnished with extra black pepper and with basil leaves, if liked.

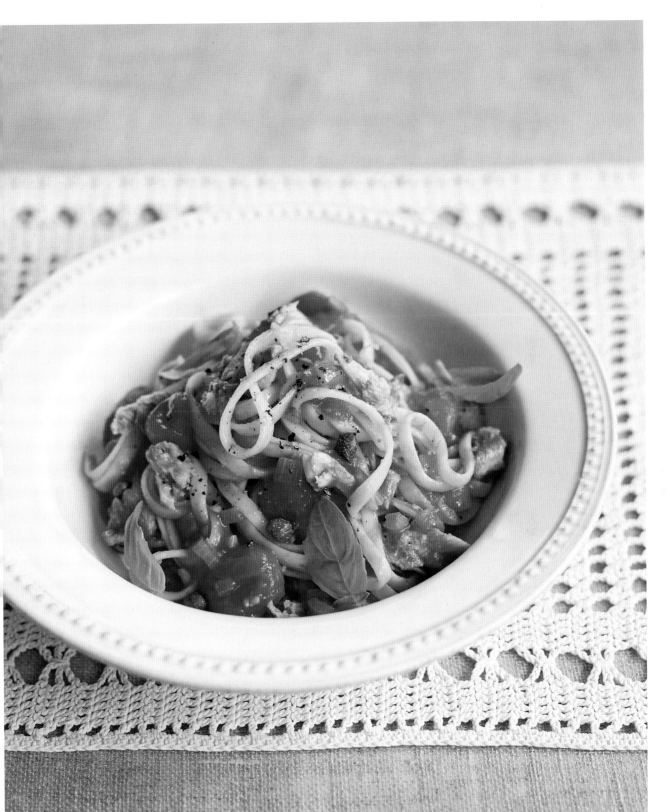

800g (1lb 12oz) floury
potatoes, peeled and diced

1 egg yolk, beaten

150g (5½oz) gluten-free
plain flour

15g (½oz) basil leaves,
finely shredded

50g (1¾oz) Parmesan
cheese, grated

4 tablespoons extra-virgin
olive oil

salt and freshly ground
black pepper

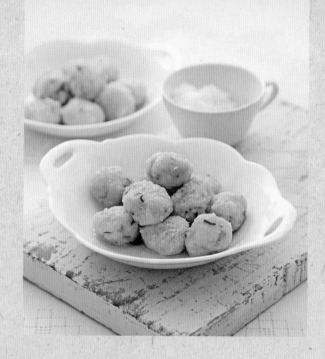

POTATO GNOCCHI

PREPARATION TIME: 20 MINUTES
COOKING TIME: 15–20 MINUTES
SERVES: 4

Cook the potatoes in a saucepan of boiling water for 12–15 minutes, until soft. Drain and mash, or use a potato ricer to obtain a really smooth texture.

Place another saucepan of water on the heat to boil.

Transfer the mashed potato to a bowl and mix in the egg yolk, flour and basil. Season with salt and pepper. Stir well to combine.

Take 1 teaspoonful of the mixture into your hand and roll it into a walnut-sized ball. Press with the tines of a fork into a gnocchi shape. Repeat with the remaining mixture.

Drop the gnocchi into the saucepan of boiling water to cook – this should take only 1–2 minutes. The gnocchi will float when cooked.

Drain and toss the hot gnocchi in the grated Parmesan and olive oil and serve immediately.

CHERRY TOMATO & PEPPER TART

Grease a baking sheet with vegetable oil and preheat the oven to 220°C (425°F), Gas Mark 7.

Roll out the pastry thinly on a lightly floured surface and cut out a 25cm (10 inch) circle. Transfer the dough circle to the prepared baking sheet. Using the tip of a sharp knife, score a continuous line around the circle 1cm (½ inch) in from the edge of the pastry to form a border.

Mix the pesto in a bowl with the tomatoes, peppers and feta. Spread the mixture in an even layer over the pastry, ensuring the filling is contained within the scored rim. Season with salt and pepper.

Place the baking sheet on the upper rack of the oven and cook for 20 minutes, until the pastry is puffed and golden, covering the tart with kitchen foil if the pastry starts to brown too much. Serve scattered with basil leaves to garnish.

PREPARATION TIME: 10 MINUTES
COOKING TIME: 25 MINUTES
SERVES: 4

vegetable oil, for greasing

375g (13oz) ready-made gluten-free puff pastry

gluten-free plain flour, for dusting

4 tablespoons Low-FODMAP Pesto (see below)

200g (7oz) cherry tomatoes, halved

150g (5½oz) mixed roasted peppers (if using ready-made, ensure the product is free from garlic), roughly chopped

100g (3½oz) feta cheese, crumbled

salt and freshly ground black pepper

basil leaves, to garnish

LOW-FODMAP PESTO

Shop-bought pesto contains garlic and is off-limits when following a low-FODMAP diet. The recipe below produces a tasty homemade alternative.

Put 50g (1¾oz) basil leaves, 3 tablespoons of pine nuts, 1 tablespoon of garlic-infused olive oil, 80ml (2¾fl oz) extra-virgin olive oil and some salt and pepper into the bowl of a food processor and process until fairly smooth. Transfer to a bowl, stir in 2 tablespoons of freshly grated Parmesan cheese and adjust the seasoning to taste.

4 chicken breasts, about
125g (4½oz) each
....

25g (1oz) basil leaves
....

2 tablespoons garlic-infused
olive oil
....

2 tablespoons pine nuts,
toasted
....

2 tablespoons grated
Parmesan cheese
....

25g (1oz) rocket, plus extra
to serve
....

800ml (1⅓ pints) boiling
water
....

200g (7oz) polenta
....

salt and freshly ground
black pepper

CHICKEN
WITH PESTO & POLENTA

PREPARATION TIME: 15 MINUTES
COOKING TIME: 10 MINUTES
SERVES: 4

Preheat the grill on the highest setting.

Slice each chicken breast in half horizontally through the middle and season all 8 pieces. Place the pieces on a grill tray.

Put the basil, oil, pine nuts, Parmesan and rocket into the bowl of a food processor or blender and process until finely chopped. Set aside.

Cook the chicken under the hot grill for 5–7 minutes, until just cooked through and still succulent.

Meanwhile, lightly salt the measured boiling water in a saucepan and stir in the polenta. Cook over medium heat, stirring constantly, for about 2 minutes, until thickened. Stir the rocket pesto through the polenta.

Serve the chicken slices on top of the polenta alongside the extra rocket leaves.

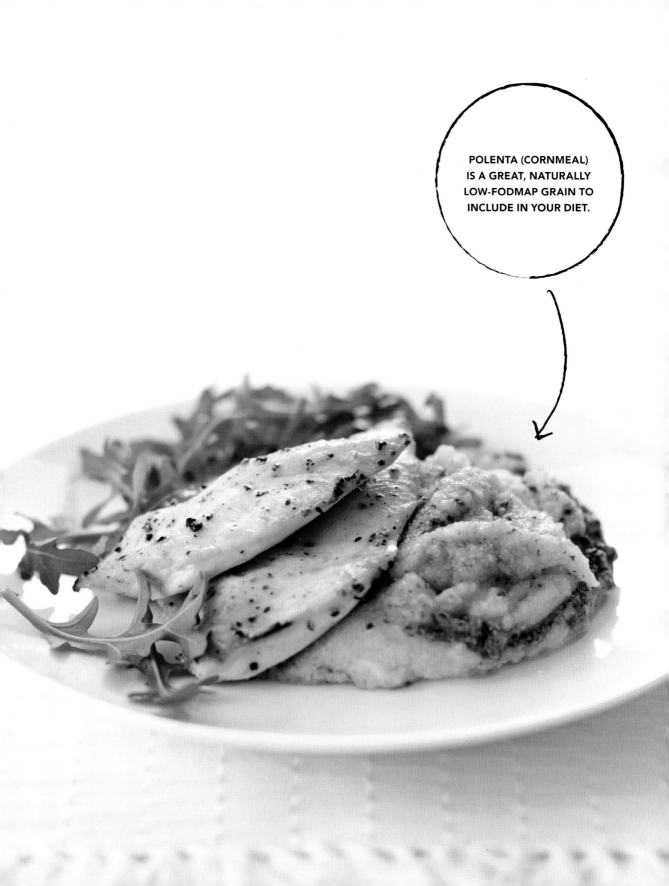

POLENTA (CORNMEAL)
IS A GREAT, NATURALLY
LOW-FODMAP GRAIN TO
INCLUDE IN YOUR DIET.

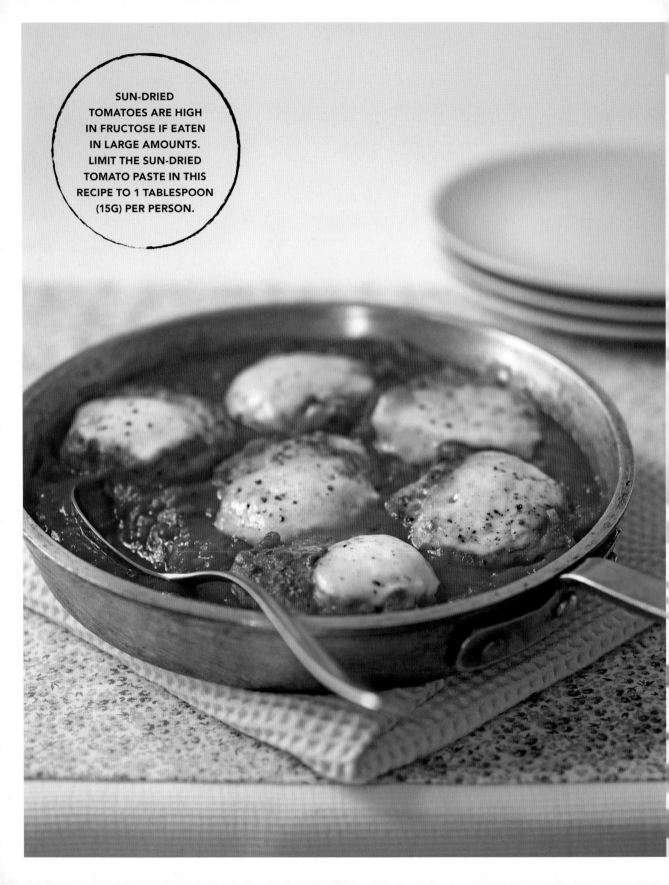

SUN-DRIED TOMATOES ARE HIGH IN FRUCTOSE IF EATEN IN LARGE AMOUNTS. LIMIT THE SUN-DRIED TOMATO PASTE IN THIS RECIPE TO 1 TABLESPOON (15G) PER PERSON.

500g (1lb 2oz) minced turkey

handful of fresh chives, snipped

50g (1¾oz) can anchovy fillets, drained and chopped

50g (1¾oz) fresh gluten-free breadcrumbs

4 tablespoons olive oil

2 x 400g (14oz) cans chopped tomatoes

2 tablespoons sun-dried tomato paste

2 teaspoons dried oregano

1 bunch of spring onions (green parts only), sliced

1 tablespoon light muscovado sugar

125g (4oz) mozzarella cheese, thinly sliced

salt and freshly ground black pepper

warmed gluten-free crusty bread, to serve (optional)

TURKEY POLPETTES
WITH TOMATOES

PREPARATION TIME: 15 MINUTES
COOKING TIME: 30 MINUTES
SERVES: 4

Mix together the turkey, chives, anchovies, breadcrumbs and a little salt and pepper in a bowl. Divide the mixture into 8 portions and shape each of these into a flat patty.

Heat 2 tablespoons of the oil in a large ovenproof frying pan. Add the patties and fry for 8 minutes, until golden on both sides. Transfer to a plate.

Add the remaining oil to the same frying pan. Stir in the tomatoes, tomato paste, oregano, spring onions, sugar and a little salt and pepper and bring to a simmer.

Return the patties to the pan, pushing them down into the sauce. Cook gently, uncovered, for 15 minutes, until the patties are cooked through.

Meanwhile, preheat the grill on a medium setting.

Place the mozzarella slices on top of the mixture in the frying pan and season with plenty of pepper. Transfer the pan to the grill and cook until the cheese melts. Serve with warmed gluten-free crusty bread, if liked.

3 tablespoons chopped mixed herbs (such as chives, parsley, rosemary and oregano)

1 tablespoon garlic-infused olive oil

finely grated zest of 1 lemon

4 thick fillets of white fish (such as cod, haddock, pollack or coley), about 150g (5½oz) each

1kg (2lb 4oz) floury potatoes, peeled and cut into chunks

2 tablespoons lemon juice

50g (1¾oz) Parmesan cheese, grated

4 tablespoons olive oil

salt and freshly ground black pepper

steamed green beans, to serve (limit each portion to 85g/3oz)

LEMON GRILLED FISH
WITH CHEESY MASHED POTATO

PREPARATION TIME: 20 MINUTES
COOKING TIME: 30 MINUTES
SERVES: 4

Mix 1 tablespoon of the chopped herbs with the garlic-infused oil, lemon zest and a little seasoning, then massage the mixture into the fish fillets. Marinate for 10–15 minutes.

Meanwhile, cook the potatoes in a large saucepan of lightly salted boiling water for 12–15 minutes, or until tender.

Heat a griddle pan until hot. Add the fish fillets with their skin sides facing downwards and cook for 4–5 minutes, until the skin is crispy. Turn the fish over, turn off the heat and set aside for 3–4 minutes, until the fish is cooked. Keep warm.

Drain the potatoes, then return them to the pan and set it over gentle heat. Allow to steam for 1–2 minutes to dry out the potatoes. Add the lemon juice, Parmesan cheese, remaining herbs, the remaining garlic-infused oil and the olive oil. Season to taste and mash until smooth, then spoon on to 4 warmed plates. Serve the cheesy mash with the grilled fish and some steamed green beans.

750g (1lb 10oz) Maris Piper
potatoes, thinly sliced

6 tablespoons olive oil

1 tablespoon chopped thyme

4 sea bream fillets, about
150g (5½oz) each

75g (2¾oz) prosciutto, chopped

1 bunch of spring onions
(green parts only), finely
chopped

finely grated zest of 1 lemon

200g (7oz) samphire

salt and freshly ground
black pepper

STUFFED BREAM WITH SAMPHIRE

PREPARATION TIME: 20 MINUTES
COOKING TIME: 55 MINUTES
SERVES: 4

Preheat the oven to 190°C (375°F), Gas Mark 5.

Toss the potato slices with 4 tablespoons of the oil, a little salt and pepper and the thyme in a bowl. Tip the mixture into a roasting tin or ovenproof dish and spread it out in an even layer. Cover the tin or dish with kitchen foil and bake for about 30 minutes, until the potatoes are tender.

Score the bream fillets several times with a sharp knife.

Mix the prosciutto with the spring onions, lemon zest and a little pepper in a bowl. Use this mixture to sandwich the bream fillets together in pairs. Tie each bundle at intervals with kitchen string. Cut each bundle of sandwiched fillets through the centre to make 4 even-sized portions.

Lay the fish over the potatoes in the baking tin and return the tin to the oven, uncovered, for a further 20 minutes or until the fish is cooked through.

Scatter the samphire around the fish and drizzle over the remaining oil. Return the tin to the oven for a further 5 minutes, then serve.

2 tablespoons garlic-infused
olive oil
....

1 bunch of spring onions
(green parts only), sliced
....

1 tablespoon tomato purée
....

400g (14oz) can chopped
tomatoes
....

pinch of sugar
....

handful of thyme leaves
....

4 skinless cod fillets, about
125g (4½oz) each
....

25g (1oz) pitted black olives
....

salt and freshly ground
black pepper
....

TO SERVE (OPTIONAL)

new potatoes
....

low-FODMAP vegetables

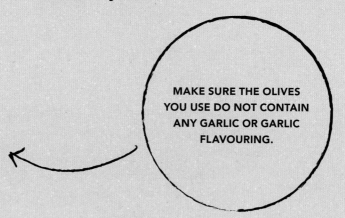

MAKE SURE THE OLIVES
YOU USE DO NOT CONTAIN
ANY GARLIC OR GARLIC
FLAVOURING.

COD IN TOMATO & OLIVE SAUCE

PREPARATION TIME: 5 MINUTES
COOKING TIME: 20–25 MINUTES
SERVES: 4

Heat the oil in a large, deep frying pan. Add the spring onions and tomato purée and cook for 1 minute over medium heat, then pour over the tomatoes. Add the sugar and thyme and season, then reduce the heat and simmer for 10 minutes.

Slide the fish fillets into the sauce along with the olives, cover loosely with kitchen foil and simmer for 8–10 minutes, until the fish flakes easily. Serve with some boiled new potatoes and your choice of low-FODMAP vegetables, if liked.

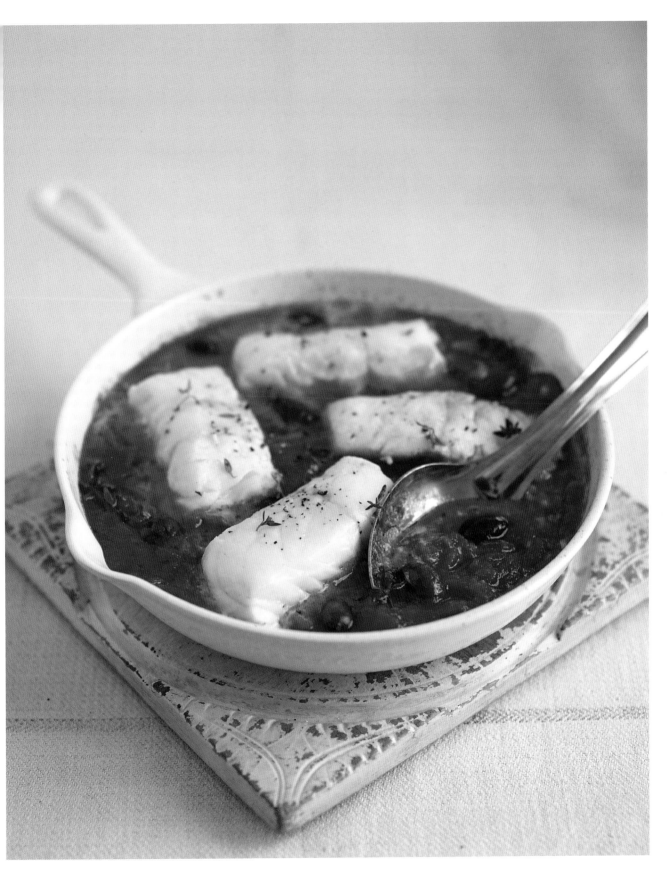

250g (9oz) brown rice

1 aubergine, cut into chunks

3 courgettes, cut into chunks

4 tablespoons flat-leaf parsley, chopped, plus extra to serve

1 tablespoon rosemary, chopped

150ml (¼ pint) olive oil

grated zest and juice of 2 lemons

250g (9oz) cherry tomatoes

100g (3½oz) blanched peanuts

2 carrots, peeled and grated

2 tablespoons light soy sauce

freshly ground black pepper

LIMIT PEANUTS TO A SMALL HANDFUL PER PORTION TO ENSURE THIS DISH REMAINS LOW FODMAP.

LEMON MIXED VEGETABLE KEBABS
WITH NUT PILAF

PREPARATION TIME: 20 MINUTES
COOKING TIME: 15 MINUTES
SERVES: 4

Cook the rice according to the packet instructions. Drain and refresh under cold running water, then drain again.

Meanwhile, preheat the grill on the highest setting. Soak 8 wooden skewers in water.

Place the aubergine and courgettes in a large bowl. Put the parsley and rosemary into a jug with the olive oil, lemon zest and juice and whisk together. Season with pepper, then pour the mixture over the vegetables and toss together.

Thread the dressed vegetables with the tomatoes on to 8 wooden skewers. Cook the skewers under the hot grill (alternatively, cook them over a barbecue), turning occasionally, for 8–10 minutes, until lightly charred and tender.

Toss the cooled rice with the peanuts, carrots, the remaining parsley and the soy sauce. Season with a little pepper. Serve the hot kebabs on a bed of the rice salad.

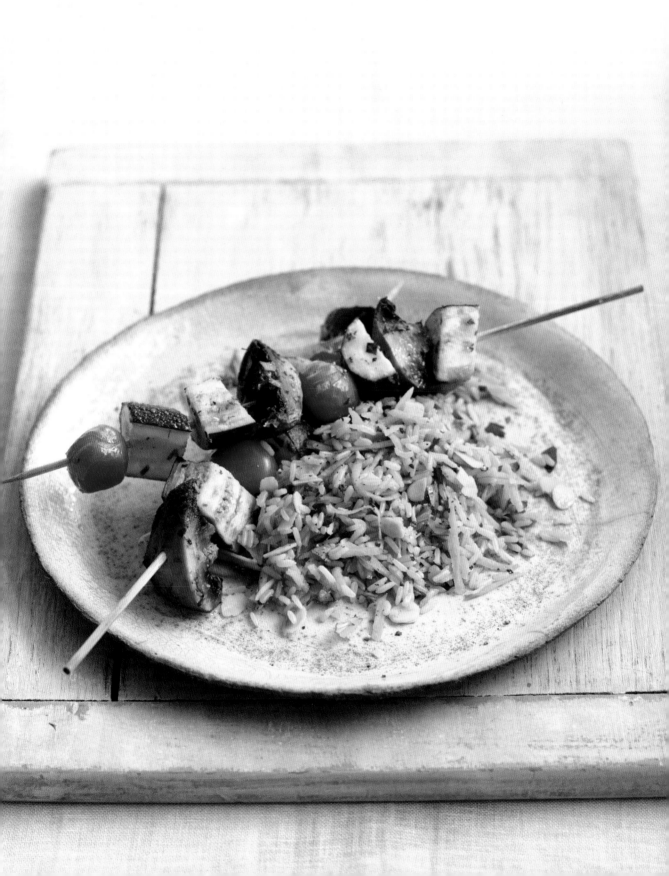

SALMON
WITH LIME COURGETTES

PREPARATION TIME: 15 MINUTES
COOKING TIME: 15–20 MINUTES
SERVES: 4

4 salmon fillets, about 150g
(5¹⁄₂oz) each

1 tablespoon English mustard

2 teaspoons peeled and
grated fresh root ginger

2 teaspoons maple syrup

1 tablespoon light soy sauce

FOR THE LIME COURGETTES

500g (1lb 2oz) courgettes,
thinly sliced lengthways

2 tablespoons olive oil

grated zest and juice of
1 lime

2 tablespoons chopped mint

salt and freshly ground
black pepper

Preheat the grill on the highest setting.

Place the salmon fillets, with their skin sides facing downwards, in a shallow ovenproof dish, ensuring they fit in the dish snugly in a single layer.

Mix the mustard, ginger, maple syrup and soy sauce in a bowl, then spoon this mixture evenly over the fillets.

Make the lime courgettes. Heat a ridged frying pan. Put the courgettes and oil into a plastic bag and toss together, then lift out the courgette slices and fry over medium heat for about 5 minutes, until lightly browned on each side and tender. You may need to do this in batches.

Stir the lime zest and juice, mint and seasoning together in a bowl.

While the courgettes are cooking, grill the salmon fillets for 10–15 minutes, depending on their thickness, until lightly charred on top and cooked through.

Transfer the salmon fillets to serving plates. Arrange the courgette slices around the fish and drizzle the lime dressing over the courgettes. Serve hot.

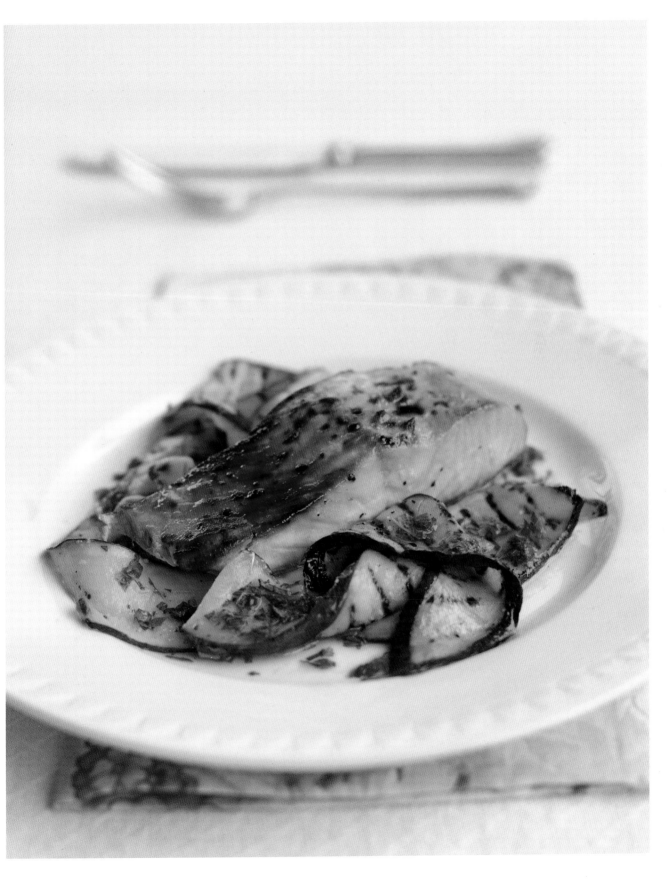

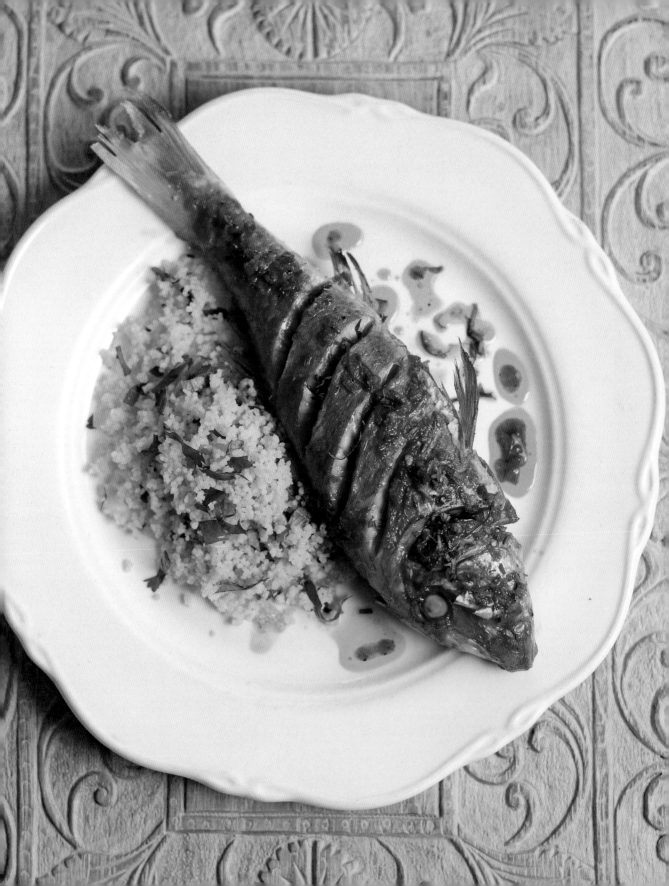

oil, for greasing

4 whole red mullet, about
125g (4½oz) each

small bunch of flat-leaf
parsley, roughly chopped,
to garnish

gluten-free couscous,
to serve

FOR THE CHERMOULA SAUCE

1 teaspoon saffron threads

2 teaspoons water

1 red chilli, deseeded
and chopped

1–2 teaspoons cumin seeds

1 teaspoon sea salt

4 tablespoons garlic-infused
olive oil

4 tablespoons lemon juice

small bunch of fresh
coriander, finely chopped

handful of chives, chopped

freshly ground black pepper

GRILLED RED MULLET FILLETS
WITH CHERMOULA SAUCE

**PREPARATION TIME: 15 MINUTES,
PLUS SOAKING
COOKING TIME: 10 MINUTES
SERVES: 4**

Preheat the grill on the highest setting. Grease a grill pan with oil.

Make the sauce first. Place the saffron in a small bowl with the measured water and leave to soak for 5 minutes.

Using a pestle and mortar, pound the chilli, cumin seeds and salt to form a coarse paste, then gradually whisk in the oil and lemon juice, then stir in the coriander and chives and season with pepper. Tip in the saffron water and mix well.

Make 3–4 slashes on both sides of each fish. Place the fish on the prepared grill pan and brush with a little of the sauce. Cook under the hot grill for 4–5 minutes, then turn, brush with a little more of the sauce and cook for 3–4 minutes, or until cooked through.

Meanwhile, heat the remaining sauce in a small saucepan. Place the fish in a serving dish, spoon over the sauce and garnish with the parsley. Serve with couscous.

SIDE DISHES

50g (1¾oz) butter

1kg (2lb 4oz) whole baby carrots, or young carrots, quartered lengthways

generous pinch of sugar

juice of 1 orange

salt and freshly ground black pepper

flat-leaf parsley, roughly chopped, to garnish

GLAZED BABY CARROTS

PREPARATION TIME: 5 MINUTES
COOKING TIME: 15–20 MINUTES
SERVES: 6

Melt the butter in a saucepan. Add the carrots and sugar and season with salt and pepper. Pour in just enough water to cover the carrots and cook gently, uncovered, for 10–12 minutes or until the carrots are tender and the liquid has evaporated. As the water evaporates, add the orange juice.

Serve garnished with chopped parsley.

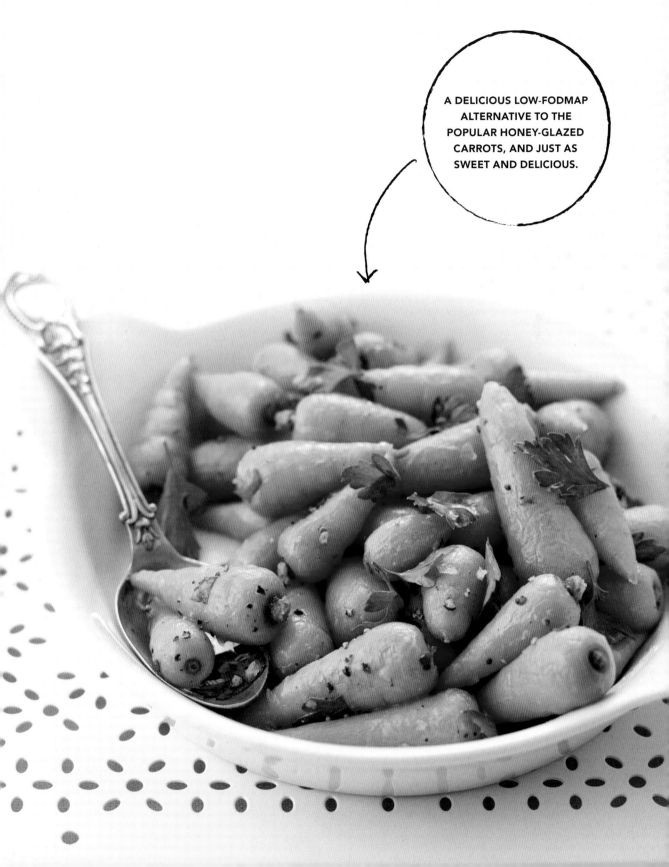

A DELICIOUS LOW-FODMAP ALTERNATIVE TO THE POPULAR HONEY-GLAZED CARROTS, AND JUST AS SWEET AND DELICIOUS.

4 baking potatoes, 175–250g
(6–9oz) each, peeled and
halved lengthways

....

4 tablespoons olive oil

....

2 tablespoons sesame seeds

....

salt

SESAME ROAST POTATOES

PREPARATION TIME: 10 MINUTES
COOKING TIME: 1–1¼ HOURS
SERVES: 4

Preheat the oven to 200°C (400°F), Gas Mark 6.

Place the potatoes on your chopping board with the cut sides facing downwards. Using a sharp knife, make cuts at 5mm (¼ inch) intervals along the length of each piece of potato, almost through to the base, so that they just hold together.

Heat the oil in a roasting tin in the oven until hot. Add the potatoes to the tin and spoon over the oil evenly. Sprinkle the potatoes with a little salt, baste well and roast for 30 minutes.

After the cooking time has elapsed, remove the potatoes from the oven and sprinkle with the sesame seeds. Return the tin to the oven and bake for a further 30 minutes or until the potatoes are golden brown and crisp.

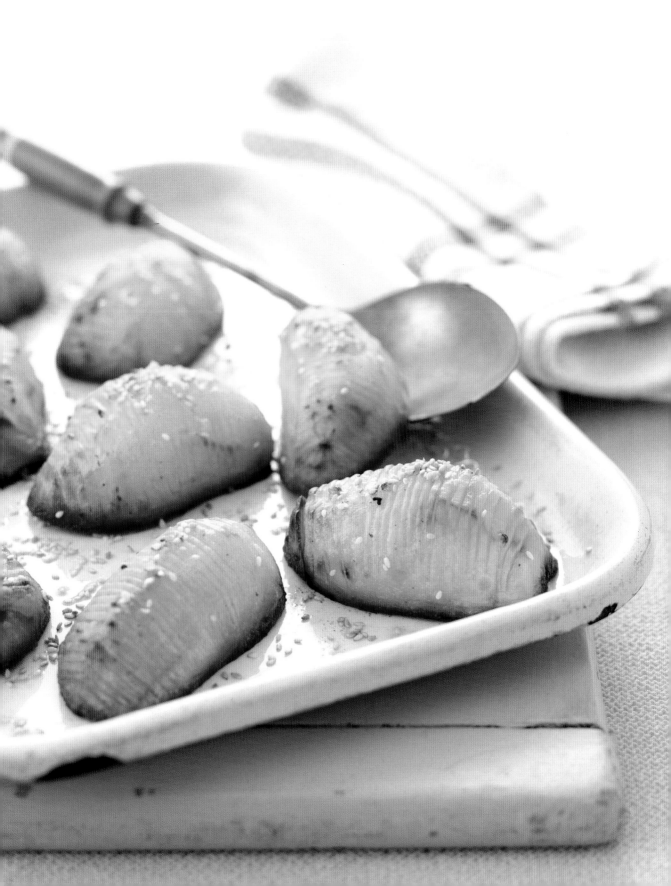

- 3 tablespoons ghee or butter
- 4 tablespoons finely chopped fresh coriander, plus extra to garnish
- rind of 1 preserved lemon, finely sliced
- 1kg (2lb 4oz) potatoes, peeled and finely sliced
- salt and freshly ground black pepper

ROASTED CORIANDER & PRESERVED LEMON POTATOES

PREPARATION TIME: 10 MINUTES
COOKING TIME: 25 MINUTES
SERVES: 4

Preheat the oven to 200°C (400°F), Gas Mark 6.

Melt the ghee or butter in a small saucepan and stir in the coriander and preserved lemon rind.

Put the potatoes into a large bowl, pour over the melted mixture and toss the potatoes well to coat.

Spread the coated potatoes in an ovenproof dish, season and cover the dish with kitchen foil. Bake for 15 minutes, then remove the foil and return the dish to the oven for a further 10 minutes, until the potatoes are tender and lightly browned.

Garnish with the extra coriander and serve alongside roasted or grilled meat, poultry or fish.

625g (1lb 6oz) baby parsnips, scrubbed

1 tablespoon garlic-infused olive oil

2 sprigs of thyme, leaves picked and chopped

1 teaspoon grated lemon zest

pinch of cayenne pepper

pinch of sea salt

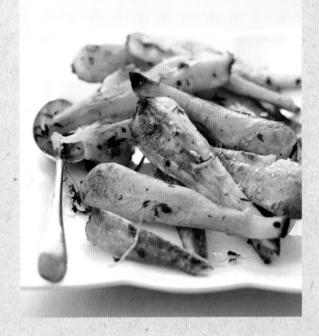

ROAST PARSNIPS
WITH THYME BUTTER

PREPARATION TIME: 10 MINUTES
COOKING TIME: 40–45 MINUTES
SERVES: 4

Preheat the oven to 200°C (400°F), Gas Mark 6.

Put all the ingredients into a large bowl and toss to coat the parsnips in the seasoned oil. Transfer to a roasting tin. Bake for 40–45 minutes, stirring occasionally, until golden and tender. Serve immediately.

100ml (3½fl oz) olive oil

1 bunch of spring onions
(green parts only), sliced

1 aubergine, cut into
bite-sized cubes

2 large courgettes, cut
into bite-sized pieces

1 red pepper, deseeded and
cut into bite-sized pieces

1 yellow pepper, deseeded
and cut into bite-sized pieces

400g (14oz) can chopped
tomatoes

4 tablespoons chopped
flat-leaf parsley or basil

salt and freshly ground
black pepper

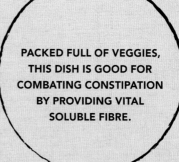

PACKED FULL OF VEGGIES,
THIS DISH IS GOOD FOR
COMBATING CONSTIPATION
BY PROVIDING VITAL
SOLUBLE FIBRE.

QUICK ONE-POT RATATOUILLE

PREPARATION TIME: 10 MINUTES
COOKING TIME: 20 MINUTES
SERVES: 4

Heat the oil in a large saucepan until very hot. Add the spring onions, aubergine, courgettes and peppers and cook over medium heat, stirring constantly, for a few minutes, until the vegetables have softened. Add the tomatoes, season to taste with salt and pepper and stir well.

Reduce the heat, cover the pan tightly with a lid and simmer for 15 minutes, until all the vegetables are cooked. Remove from the heat and stir in the chopped parsley or basil before serving.

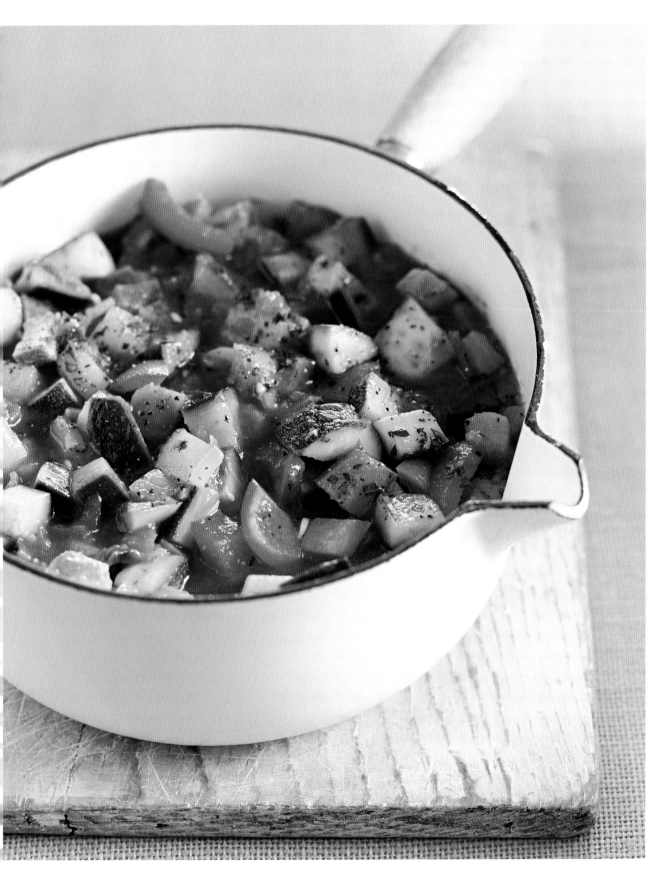

5 tablespoons garlic-infused olive oil

1 bunch of spring onions (green parts only), sliced

200g (7oz) can chopped tomatoes

1 green pepper, deseeded and sliced

1 aubergine or 3 baby aubergines, sliced

1 courgette or 4 baby courgettes, sliced

salt and freshly ground black pepper

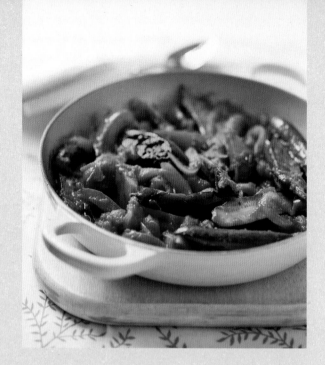

BRAISED SPANISH VEGETABLES

PREPARATION TIME: 10 MINUTES
COOKING TIME: 35 MINUTES
SERVES: 4–6

Heat 1 tablespoon of the oil in a large frying pan over medium heat. Add the spring onions and cook for 5–7 minutes, until softened. Add the tomatoes and a splash of water and simmer for 15 minutes.

Meanwhile, heat 1 tablespoon of the oil in a separate frying pan. Add the green pepper and cook for 5 minutes, stirring, until softened and lightly browned. Remove the pepper from the pan and set aside. Pour another 2 tablespoons of the oil into the pan. Add the aubergine and cook for 5 minutes, until golden, then set aside. Add the remaining oil to the pan, add the courgette and cook for 5 minutes, until golden.

Return the pepper and aubergine to the pan, pour over the tomato sauce and season well. Bring to a boil, then reduce the heat and simmer for 10 minutes, until the vegetables are very tender and most of the liquid has evaporated.

4 courgettes

175g (6oz) plum tomatoes,
chopped

210g (7½oz) mozzarella
cheese, grated

2 tablespoons shredded
basil leaves

25g (1oz) Parmesan cheese,
grated

salt and freshly ground
black pepper

STUFFED COURGETTES

PREPARATION TIME: 15 MINUTES
COOKING TIME: 30 MINUTES
SERVES: 4

Preheat the oven to 200°C (400°F), Gas Mark 6.

Slice the courgettes in half horizontally, then scoop out the centre of each half, reserving the flesh. Place the courgette halves in a roasting tin and bake for 10 minutes, until slightly softened.

Meanwhile, chop the reserved courgette flesh and mix it in a bowl with the chopped tomatoes, grated mozzarella and basil. Season with salt and pepper.

Remove the courgette halves from the oven and spoon the filling into each courgette shell. Sprinkle over the grated Parmesan and return the tin to the oven. Bake for a further 15 minutes, until golden.

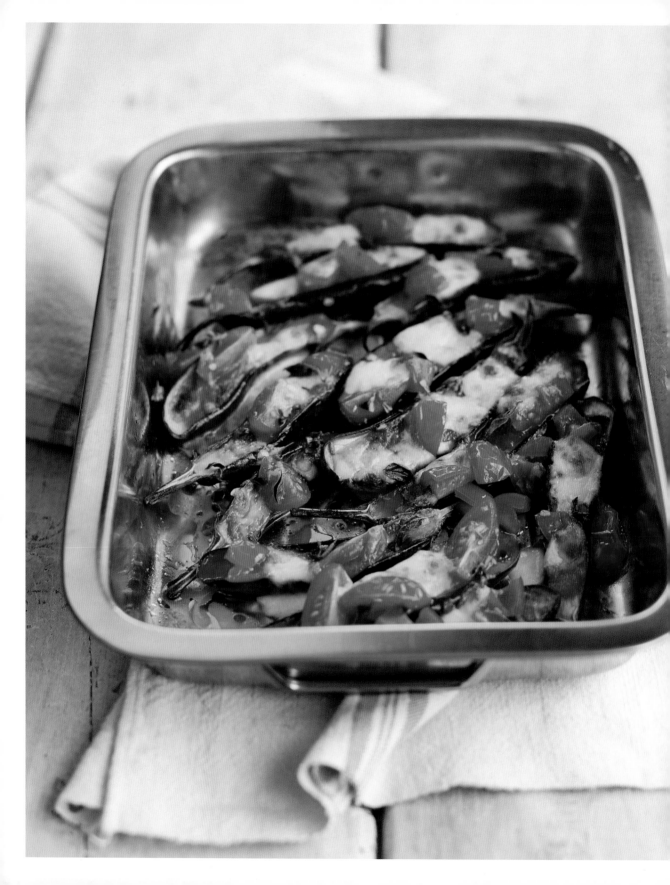

- 5 tablespoons olive oil
- 12 baby aubergines, halved
- 125ml (4fl oz) passata (free from sun-dried tomatoes)
- 75g (2¾oz) vine tomatoes, chopped
- pinch of chilli flakes
- handful of oregano leaves, chopped
- 200g (7oz) mozzarella cheese, sliced
- salt and freshly ground black pepper

THE AMOUNT OF LACTOSE IN MOZZARELLA CAN VARY, SO WHILE IN THE ELIMINATION STAGES OF THE LOW-FODMAP DIET LIMIT MOZZARELLA TO 50G (1¾OZ) PER PORTION.

AUBERGINE, TOMATO & MOZZARELLA MELTS

PREPARATION TIME: 10 MINUTES
COOKING TIME: 20 MINUTES
SERVES: 4

Preheat the grill on the highest setting.

Rub the oil over the aubergines and season well. Place them on a grill pan and cook under the hot grill for 5–7 minutes on each side or until soft and golden brown.

Mix together the passata, tomatoes, chilli and oregano and season well. Arrange the aubergines on the grill pan with their cut sides facing upwards. Spoon a little of the passata mixture on top of each aubergine half and place some mozzarella slices on top. Grill for 2–3 minutes, until the mozzarella has just melted. Serve immediately.

4 red or yellow peppers,
halved and deseeded

4 small vine tomatoes, halved

200g (7oz) feta cheese, sliced

3 spring onions (green parts
only), thinly sliced

2 tablespoons olive oil or
vegetable oil, plus extra
for greasing

250g (9oz) gluten-free
couscous

25g (1oz) butter

freshly ground black pepper

2 tablespoons pumpkin or
sunflower seeds, to garnish
(optional)

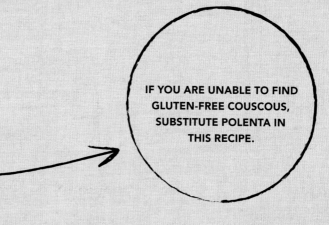

IF YOU ARE UNABLE TO FIND
GLUTEN-FREE COUSCOUS,
SUBSTITUTE POLENTA IN
THIS RECIPE.

BAKED PEPPERS
WITH FETA & SPRING ONION

PREPARATION TIME: 10 MINUTES
COOKING TIME: 25 MINUTES
SERVES: 4

Preheat the oven to 200°C (400°F), Gas Mark 6. Lightly grease a
baking sheet.

Put the pepper halves on to the prepared baking sheet with their
cut sides facing upwards. Fill the recesses with the tomato halves,
feta slices and spring onions. Season with black pepper and drizzle
with the oil. Bake for 20–25 minutes, until softened and golden.

Meanwhile, put the couscous into a bowl with the butter and pour
over 300ml (½ pint) boiling water. Cover the bowl and set aside
for 5–8 minutes, until the liquid has been absorbed and the grains
are tender.

Serve the baked peppers with the couscous, scattered with pumpkin
or sunflower seeds, if using.

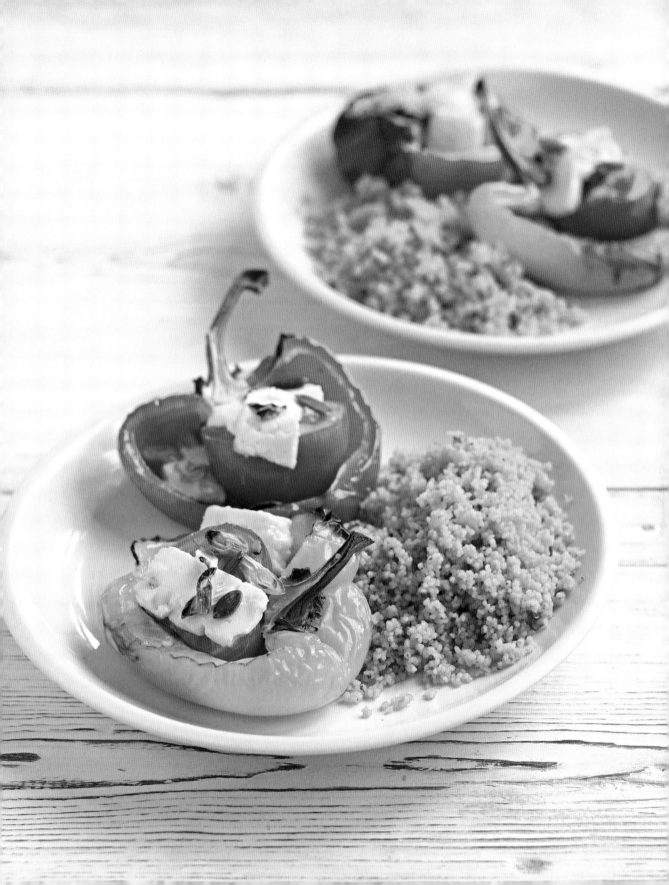

spray oil, for oiling

1 litre (1¾ pints) water

2 teaspoons salt

175g (6oz) polenta

50g (1¾oz) butter

50g (1¾oz) Parmesan cheese,
grated, plus extra to serve

olive oil, for brushing

freshly ground black pepper

chopped flat-leaf parsley,
to garnish

CHARGRILLED POLENTA TRIANGLES

**PREPARATION TIME: 10 MINUTES,
PLUS COOLING**

COOKING TIME: 15–20 MINUTES

SERVES: 8

Lightly oil a 23 x 30cm (9 x 12 inch) baking tin with spray oil.

Bring the measured water to a boil in a heavy-based saucepan. Add the salt, then gradually whisk in the polenta in a steady stream. Cook over low heat, stirring constantly with a wooden spoon, for 5 minutes, until the grains have swelled and thickened.

Remove the pan from the heat and immediately beat in the butter, Parmesan and pepper until smooth. Pour the mixture into the prepared tin and leave to cool.

Turn out the polenta on to a chopping board and cut it into large squares. Cut each square diagonally in half into triangles. Brush the triangles with a little oil.

Heat a griddle pan until hot. Add the polenta triangles, in batches, and cook over medium-high heat for 2–3 minutes on each side, until charred and heated through. Serve immediately, garnished with grated Parmesan and chopped parsley.

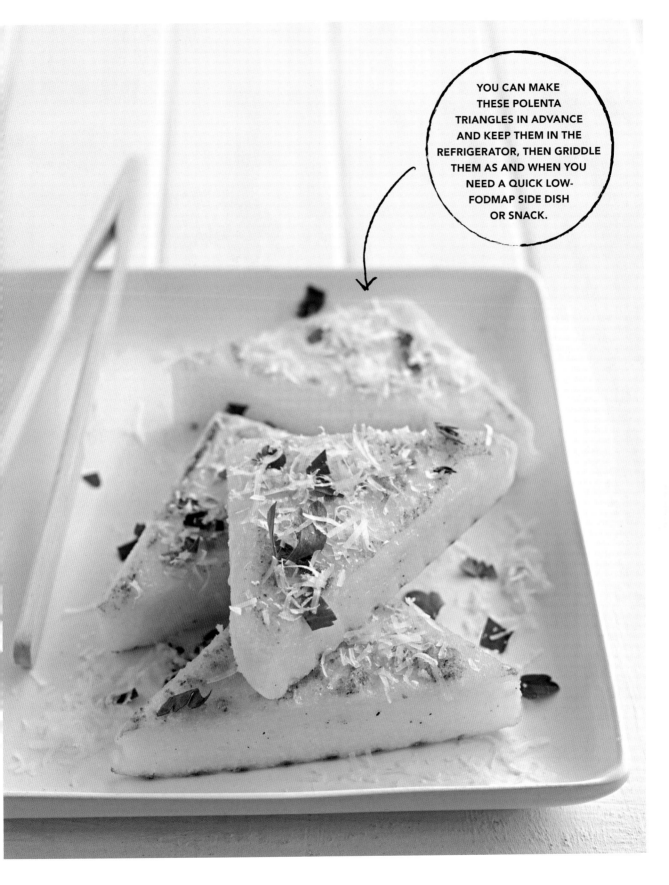

YOU CAN MAKE THESE POLENTA TRIANGLES IN ADVANCE AND KEEP THEM IN THE REFRIGERATOR, THEN GRIDDLE THEM AS AND WHEN YOU NEED A QUICK LOW-FODMAP SIDE DISH OR SNACK.

CARROT & PEPPER PILAF

PREPARATION TIME: 20 MINUTES, PLUS SOAKING AND STANDING
COOKING TIME: 20 MINUTES
SERVES: 4

275g (9¾oz) basmati rice

4 tablespoons sunflower oil

1 cinnamon stick

2 teaspoons cumin seeds

2 cloves

4 cardamom pods, lightly bruised

8 black peppercorns

1 large carrot, peeled and coarsely grated

200g (7oz) fresh or frozen sliced peppers

500ml (18fl oz) hot water

salt and freshly ground black pepper

Wash the rice several times in cold water, then leave it to soak for 15 minutes. Drain thoroughly.

Heat the oil in a heavy-based saucepan. Add the spices and stir-fry for 2–3 minutes, until they release their aromas, then add the carrot and peppers. Stir-fry for 2–3 minutes, until the vegetables are well coated in the spicy oil, then add the rice. Stir the mixture as you pour in the measured hot water. Season well.

Bring the mixture to a boil, cover the saucepan tightly with a lid, reduce the heat and simmer gently for 10 minutes. Do not lift the lid to ensure you retain the steam inside the pan, which is required for the cooking process.

Remove the pan from the heat and leave to stand, covered and undisturbed, for 8–10 minutes. Fluff up the grains with a fork and serve immediately.

1 tablespoon sunflower oil

2 aubergines, cut into cubes

1 red chilli, deseeded and thinly sliced

2 teaspoons tamarind paste

1 tablespoon dark muscovado sugar

500g (1lb 2oz) cooked basmati rice

8 tablespoons mint leaves, roughly chopped

200g (7oz) baby spinach leaves

1 bunch of spring onions (green parts only), thinly sliced

salt and freshly ground black pepper

TAMARIND CAN BE HIGH IN FODMAPS IF EATEN IN LARGER QUANTITIES, SO STICK TO THE QUANTITY STATED IN THIS RECIPE – USE NO MORE THAN ½ TEASPOON PER PORTION.

TAMARIND RICE

PREPARATION TIME: 10 MINUTES

COOKING TIME: ABOUT 15 MINUTES

SERVES: 4

Warm the oil in a large frying pan over high heat. Add the cubed aubergine, half the sliced chilli, 1 teaspoon of the tamarind paste and the muscovado sugar. Stir-fry for 5 minutes, until the aubergine is golden and beginning to soften.

Add the cooked rice, mint, spinach, spring onions and the remaining tamarind to the aubergine. Stir-fry for a further 5–6 minutes or until piping hot.

Sprinkle over the remaining chilli slices. Season with salt and pepper and serve immediately.

CAKES, BAKES & SWEET TREATS

SPICY GRIDDLED PINEAPPLE →

Heat a frying pan or griddle pan until very hot. Add the pineapple slices and cook until they start to caramelize, turning them over just once.

Add the maple syrup, chilli flakes and cinnamon and cook until the mixture starts to bubble – this will not take long.

Serve the pineapple slices drizzled with the spicy maple syrup and a dollop of yogurt.

PREPARATION TIME: 5 MINUTES
COOKING TIME: 10 MINUTES
SERVES: 4

8 slices of fresh pineapple, peeled and cored

1 tablespoon maple syrup

pinch of chilli flakes

pinch of ground cinnamon

plain lactose-free or plant-based yogurt (limit soya yogurt to 60g/2¼oz per portion), or standard yogurt if you know you tolerate lactose

ORANGE BLOSSOM & ALMOND ORANGES

PREPARATION TIME: 10 MINUTES
SERVES: 4

4 large oranges

2–3 teaspoons orange blossom water

1 tablespoon icing sugar

2 tablespoons almonds, roughly chopped

Using a sharp knife, slice the tops and bases off the oranges, then remove the skin and pith. Slice each orange into 6 rounds, reserving any juice.

Mix together the reserved juice, orange slices, orange blossom water, to taste, and icing sugar in a bowl.

Divide the orange slices between 4 bowls, then drizzle the juice over each serving. Sprinkle over the almonds to serve.

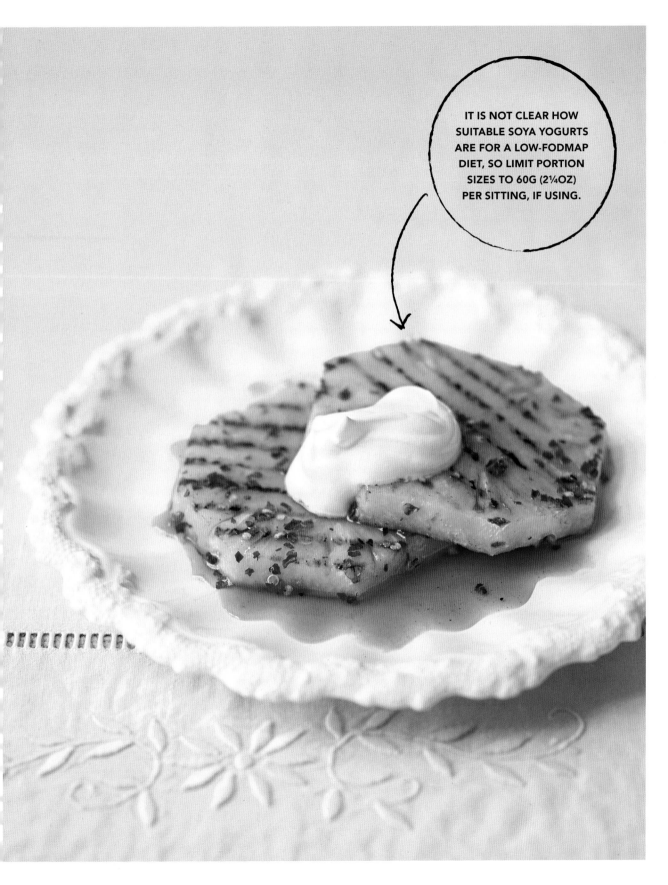

IT IS NOT CLEAR HOW SUITABLE SOYA YOGURTS ARE FOR A LOW-FODMAP DIET, SO LIMIT PORTION SIZES TO 60G (2¼OZ) PER SITTING, IF USING.

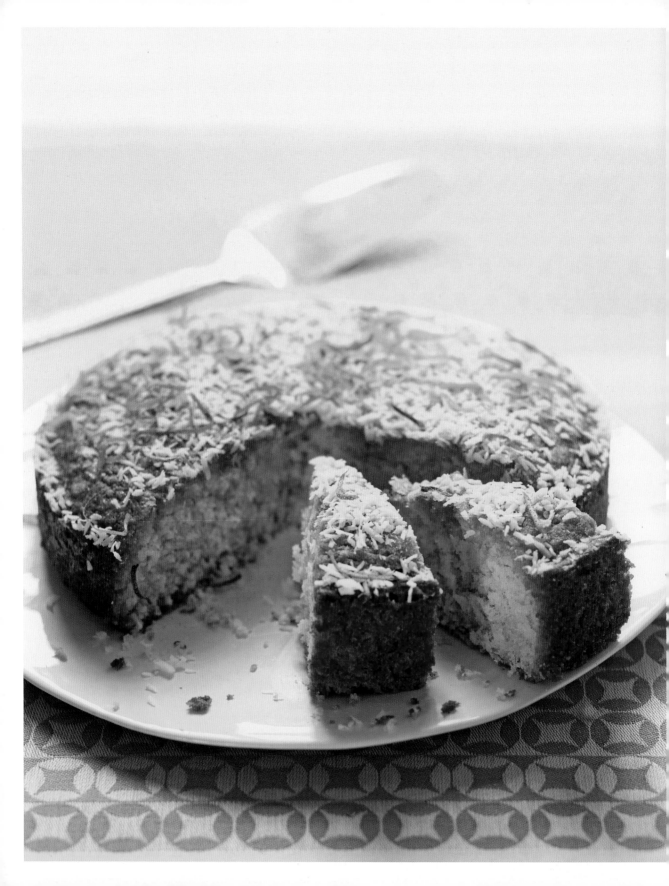

200g (7oz) unsalted butter, softened

200g (7oz) caster sugar

finely grated zest of 2 limes

3 eggs, lightly beaten

200g (7oz) gluten-free self-raising flour, sifted

50g (1¾oz) desiccated coconut

FOR THE TOPPING

4 tablespoons caster sugar

juice of 2 limes

2 tablespoons desiccated coconut or freshly grated coconut

finely pared long strands of lime rind

LIME & COCONUT DRIZZLE CAKE

PREPARATION TIME: 20 MINUTES, PLUS COOLING

COOKING TIME: 35–40 MINUTES

SERVES: 8

Preheat the oven to 180°C (350°F), Gas Mark 4. Grease a 20cm (8 inch) round springform cake tin and line the base with nonstick baking paper.

Beat the butter, sugar and grated lime zest together in a large bowl using a hand-held electric whisk until pale and fluffy. Beat in the eggs a little at a time, adding 1 tablespoon of the flour if the mixture starts to curdle, then fold in the flour and coconut with a large metal spoon.

Spoon the mixture into the prepared tin and bake in the centre of the oven for 35–40 minutes, until risen, golden and shrinking away from the tin. Leave to cool in the tin.

While the cake is still warm, make the topping. Mix the sugar with the lime juice and spoon the mixture over the cake. Sprinkle over the coconut and strands of lime rind. Leave to cool completely before removing from the tin and slicing.

200g (7oz) gluten-free flour

2 eggs

300ml (½ pint) lactose-free
or plant-based milk (limit
soya to 60ml/4 tablespoons per
portion), or standard milk if
you know you tolerate lactose

½ tablespoon sunflower oil,
for greasing

2 oranges

2–3 tablespoons caster
sugar, to serve

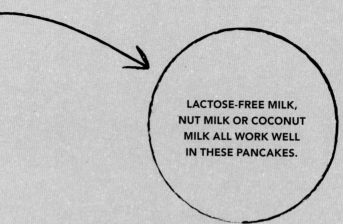

**LACTOSE-FREE MILK,
NUT MILK OR COCONUT
MILK ALL WORK WELL
IN THESE PANCAKES.**

SWEET ORANGE PANCAKES

**PREPARATION TIME: 15 MINUTES,
    PLUS STANDING
COOKING TIME: 40–60 MINUTES
SERVES: 4**

Sift the flour into a bowl and make a well in the centre. Add the eggs and whisk, using a hand-held electric whisk, while gradually adding the milk, to incorporate the flour into the batter. Leave to stand for 10 minutes.

Heat a small frying pan over medium heat. Lightly oil the pan by wiping it with an oiled piece of kitchen paper. Pour a generous tablespoonful of the batter into the pan and roll it around to completely coat the base of the pan. Cook for 3–4 minutes, then turn over and cook the other side for 2–3 minutes, until pale golden. Transfer the pancake to a sheet of baking paper and keep warm. Repeat with the remaining batter to make 8 pancakes.

Grate the orange zest, then segment the oranges, catching the juice. Pour the juice into another pan, add the segments and zest and warm through. Divide the mixture into 8 portions and pour 1 of these over each pancake, then sprinkle over some caster sugar to serve.

**PREPARATION TIME: 10 MINUTES,
PLUS MARINATING
COOKING TIME: 5–10 MINUTES
SERVES: 4**

juice of 2 limes

6 tablespoons caster sugar

4 bananas, sliced into
3–4 pieces

200g (7oz) cornflour

100g (3½oz) gluten-free
self-raising flour

3 tablespoons desiccated
coconut

3 large egg yolks

75ml (2½fl oz) chilled soda
water or sparkling water

vegetable oil, for deep-frying

icing sugar, for dusting

maple syrup, for drizzling

LIME, BANANA &
COCONUT FRITTERS

Preheat the oven to 150°C (300°F), Gas Mark 2.

Mix together the lime juice and caster sugar in a
bowl. Add the bananas, stir well to coat and leave
to marinate for 5 minutes.

Roll the bananas in half the cornflour until well
coated and set aside.

Sift the remaining cornflour and self-raising flour
into a bowl. Stir in the coconut.

Whisk together the egg yolks and soda or sparkling
water in a clean bowl. Add the flour mixture and
whisk again until the mixture forms a thick batter.

Fill a deep medium-sized saucepan one-quarter
full of vegetable oil. Heat the oil to 180°C (350°F)
or until a cube of bread immersed in the oil turns
golden in 10–15 seconds.

Dip each piece of banana in the batter and
carefully place it in the hot vegetable oil. Deep-fry
in batches, for 1–2 minutes, until golden brown.
Carefully remove the fritters from the oil using
a slotted spoon and drain on kitchen paper. Keep
the fritters warm on a plate in the warm oven while
you fry the rest.

Serve immediately, dusted with icing sugar and
drizzled with maple syrup.

250g (9oz) strawberries, hulled and roughly chopped

1 teaspoon finely grated lemon zest

1–2 teaspoons maple syrup, to taste

$\frac{1}{2}$ teaspoon vanilla bean paste or extract

2 teaspoons finely chopped mint (optional)

1 large egg white

50g (1$\frac{3}{4}$oz) caster sugar

DON'T HAVE MORE THAN 1 SERVING OF THIS DISH AT A TIME TO REMAIN WITHIN THE FODMAP THRESHOLD – YOU SHOULD CONSUME NO MORE THAN 80G (2¾OZ) FRUIT PER SITTING.

INDIVIDUAL BAKED STRAWBERRY & LEMON MERINGUES

PREPARATION TIME: 20 MINUTES
COOKING TIME: 5–7 MINUTES
SERVES: 4

Preheat the oven to 200°C (400°F), Gas Mark 6.

Put the strawberries, lemon zest, maple syrup, vanilla bean paste and chopped mint into a bowl and toss until all the ingredients are well combined. Spoon the strawberries and any liquid into 4 ramekins or other small, ovenproof dishes.

Place the egg white in a large, clean bowl and use a hand-held electric whisk to whisk it to firm peaks. Add the sugar, a tablespoon at a time, whisking constantly, until all the sugar has been incorporated.

Spoon the raw meringue mixture in a high peak into each ramekin over the fruit, then bake for 5–7 minutes or until pale golden. Remove from the oven and serve immediately.

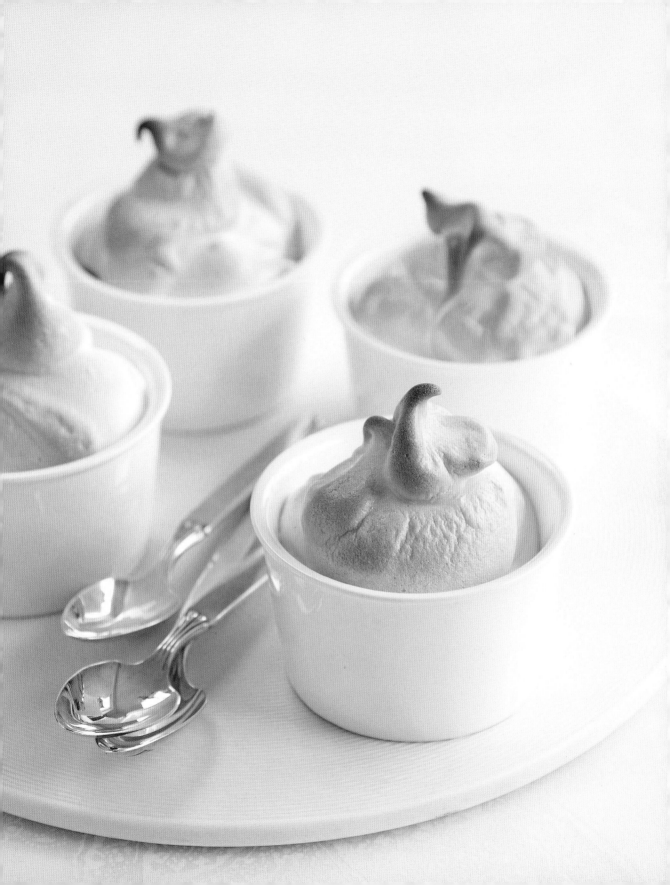

MELON, GINGER & LIME SORBET

PREPARATION TIME: 15 MINUTES, PLUS CHURNING AND FREEZING

SERVES: 4

1 large ripe Charentais melon or Galia melon, chilled
....
150g (5½oz) caster sugar
....
1 tablespoon peeled and finely grated fresh root ginger
....
juice of 2 limes
....
ice cream wafers, to serve

Cut the melon in half, remove and discard the seeds, then roughly chop the flesh – you need about 450g (1lb). Place it in a food processor with the sugar, ginger and lime juice and blend until smooth.

Transfer the sorbet to an ice cream maker and process according to the manufacturer's instructions. Alternatively, if you don't have an ice cream maker, place the mixture in a freezer-proof container and freeze for about 2–3 hours or until ice crystals have appeared on the surface. Beat with a hand-held electric whisk until smooth, then return the mixture to the freezer. Repeat this process twice more until you have a fine-textured sorbet, then freeze until firm.

Remove the sorbet from the freezer 10 minutes before serving. Serve scooped into glasses, with a wafer.

150g (5½oz) butter, softened

150g (5½oz) caster sugar

75g (2¾oz) rice flour

75g (2¾oz) cornflour

1 tablespoon baking powder

grated zest and juice of
1 lemon

3 eggs, beaten

125g (4½oz) raspberries

1 tablespoon lemon curd
(free from added fructose)

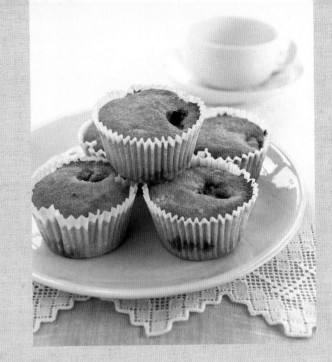

LEMON & RASPBERRY CUPCAKES

**PREPARATION TIME: 15 MINUTES,
PLUS COOLING**
COOKING TIME: 12–15 MINUTES
MAKES: 12

Preheat the oven to 200°C (400°F), Gas Mark 6. Line a large 12-hole muffin tin with paper muffin cases.

Whisk together all the ingredients, except the raspberries and the lemon curd, in a large bowl. Fold in the raspberries.

Spoon half the sponge mixture into the prepared muffin cases. Dot over a little of the lemon curd, then add the remaining mixture.

Bake for 12–15 minutes, until golden and firm to the touch. Remove from the oven, transfer to a wire rack and leave to cool.

225g (8oz) gluten-free
self-raising flour

1 teaspoon gluten-free
baking powder

½ teaspoon bicarbonate
of soda

75g (2¾oz) caster sugar

40g (1½oz) desiccated coconut

55g (2oz) unsalted butter,
melted

2 eggs

150ml (¼ pint) lactose-free
or plant-based milk (limit
soya to 60ml/4 tablespoons per
portion), or standard milk if
you know you tolerate lactose

125g (4½oz) raspberries

YOU CAN USE FROZEN RASPBERRIES FOR THIS RECIPE IF FRESH BERRIES ARE OUT OF SEASON.

COCONUT & RASPBERRY MUFFINS

PREPARATION TIME: 10 MINUTES,
**   PLUS COOLING**
COOKING TIME: 15 MINUTES
MAKES: 12

Preheat the oven to 200°C (400°F), Gas Mark 6. Line a 12-hole muffin tin with paper muffin cases.

In a large bowl, sift together the flour, baking powder and bicarbonate of soda, then mix in the sugar and coconut. Make a well in the centre of the mixture.

Whisk together the melted butter, eggs and milk in another bowl. Pour the wet ingredients into the dry ingredients and mix together gently, then fold in the raspberries when the mixture is nearly combined – do not over mix.

Spoon the batter into the paper cases. Bake for 15 minutes, until golden and slightly risen. Cool on a wire rack.

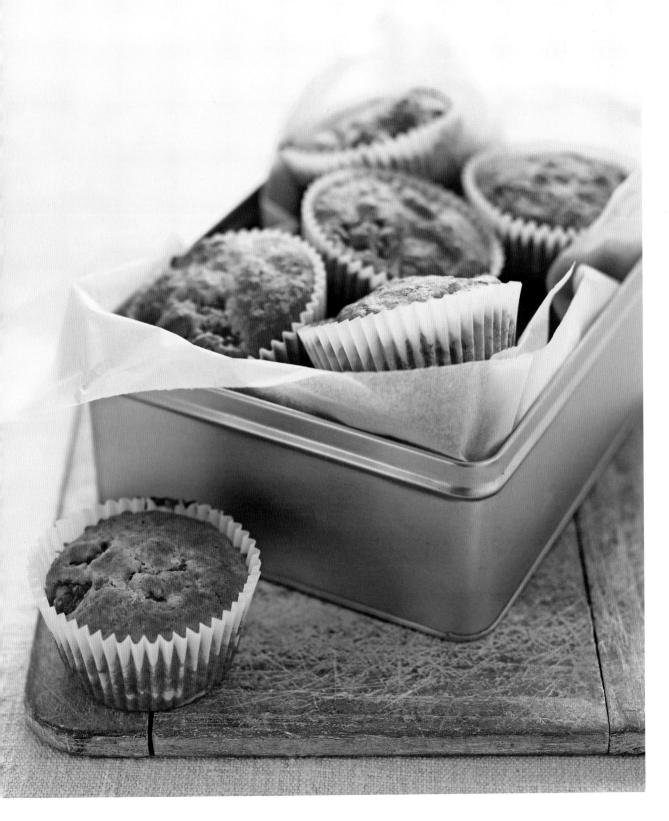

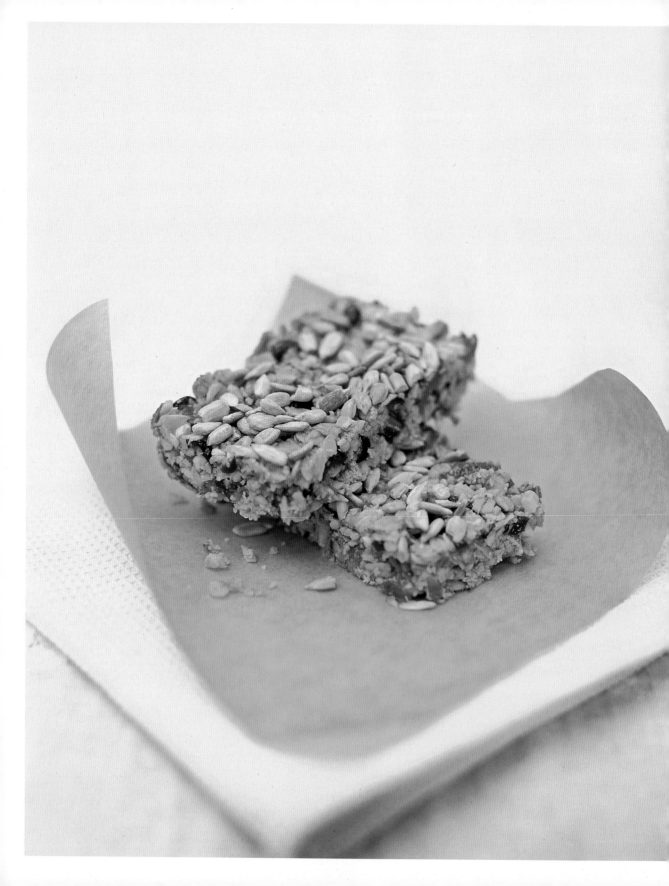

100g (3½oz) butter, plus extra for greasing

4 tablespoons maple syrup

2 tablespoons soft light brown sugar

150g (5½oz) jumbo oats

100g (3½oz) oatmeal

100g (3½oz) mixed low-FODMAP nuts (such as walnuts, peanuts and macadamia nuts), chopped

50g (1¾oz) dried blueberries

2 tablespoons sunflower seeds

IF YOU ARE FOLLOWING A GLUTEN-FREE DIET FOR COELIAC OR GLUTEN SENSITIVITY, YOU WILL NEED TO CHOOSE GLUTEN-FREE OATS.

FRUIT & NUT BARS

PREPARATION TIME: 10 MINUTES, PLUS COOLING

COOKING TIME: 18–20 MINUTES

MAKES: 8

Preheat the oven to 200°C (400°F), Gas Mark 6. Grease a 20cm (8 inch) square nonstick baking tin lightly and line the base with nonstick baking paper.

Melt the butter, syrup and sugar together in a saucepan. Stir in the remaining ingredients, except the sunflower seeds, then press the mixture into the prepared tin.

Sprinkle over the sunflower seeds, then bake for 15 minutes or until golden. Cut into 8 bars and leave to cool.

PREPARATION TIME: 20 MINUTES
COOKING TIME: 35–45 MINUTES
SERVES: 8–10

butter, for greasing

4 egg whites

1/4 teaspoon cream of tartar

125g (4 1/2 oz) light muscovado sugar

100g (3 1/2 oz) caster sugar

1 teaspoon white wine vinegar

50g (1 3/4 oz) walnut pieces, lightly toasted and chopped

FOR THE FILLING

200ml (7fl oz) whipping cream

250g (9oz) strawberries

STRAWBERRY MACAROON CAKE

Preheat the oven to 150°C (300°F), Gas Mark 2. Grease 2 x 20cm (8 inch) sandwich tins and line the bases with nonstick baking paper.

Whisk the egg whites and cream of tartar in a large clean bowl until stiff. Combine the sugars in a bowl, then gradually whisk the sugars into the egg white a little at a time, until fully incorporated. Add the vinegar and whisk for a few minutes more until the meringue mixture is thick and glossy. Fold in the walnuts.

Divide the meringue mixture evenly between the prepared sandwich tins. Level off the surfaces, then swirl the tops with the back of a spoon. Bake for 35–45 minutes, until lightly browned and crisp. Use a sharp knife to loosen the edges of the meringues in the tins, then leave to cool in the tins.

Re-loosen the edges of the meringues, then turn out each meringue on to a clean tea towel. Peel off the lining papers. Put 1 of the meringues on to a serving plate.

Whip the cream to soft peaks, then spoon three-quarters of the whipped cream over the meringue on the serving plate. Halve 8 of the smallest strawberries and set aside. Hull and slice the remaining berrries and arrange them on the layer of cream. Cover with the second meringue, ensuring the top of this meringue layer is facing upwards. Decorate with spoonfuls of the remaining cream and the reserved halved strawberries. Serve within 2 hours of assembly.

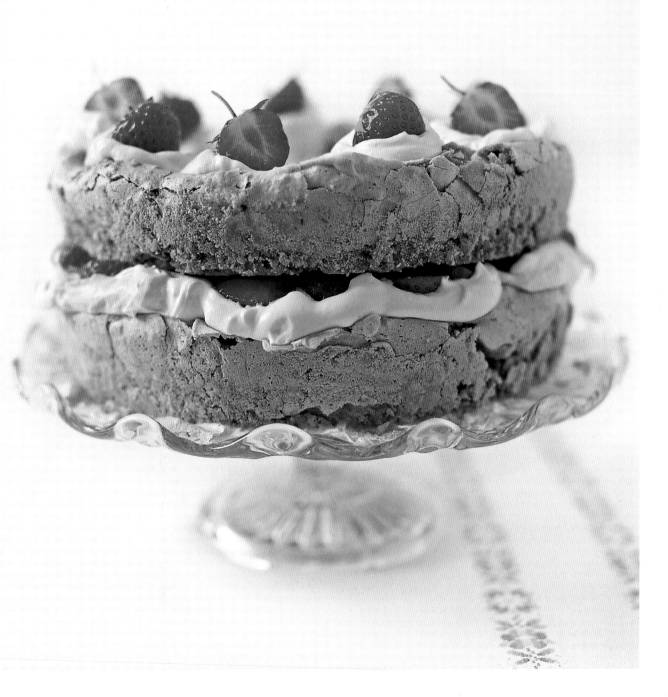

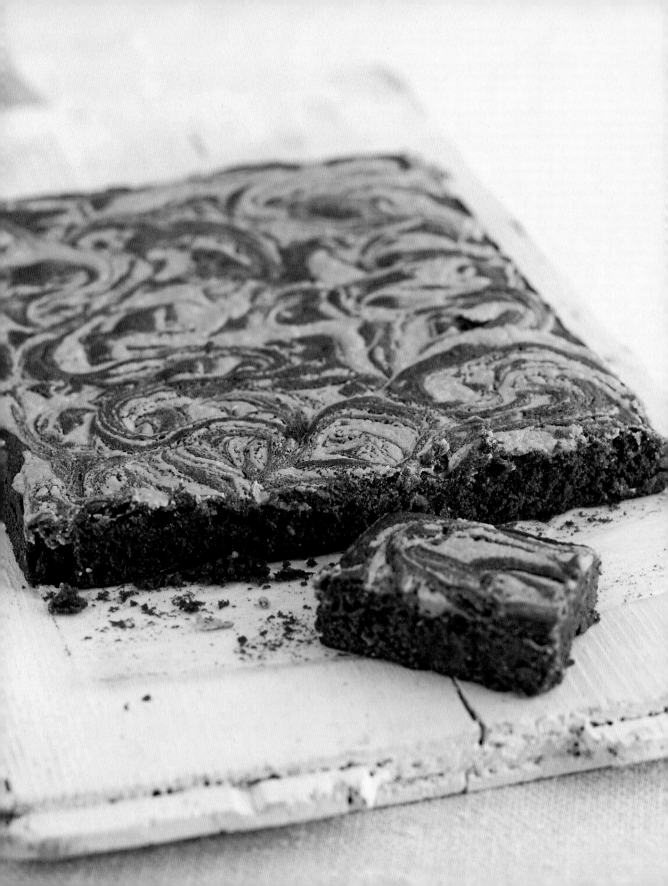

- 175g (6oz) unsalted butter, plus extra for greasing
- 200g (7oz) plain dark chocolate, broken into small pieces
- 75g (3oz) crunchy peanut butter (free from high-fructose corn syrup)
- 125g (4$\frac{1}{2}$oz) smooth peanut butter (free from high-fructose corn syrup)
- 3 large eggs
- 175g (6oz) caster sugar
- $\frac{1}{4}$ teaspoon salt
- 50g (1$\frac{3}{4}$oz) gluten-free self-raising flour

PEANUT BUTTER SWIRL BROWNIES

PREPARATION TIME: 10 MINUTES
COOKING TIME: 30 MINUTES
MAKES: 12–16

Preheat the oven to 200°C (400°F), Gas Mark 6. Grease a 30 x 20cm (12 x 8 inch) brownie tin and line it with nonstick baking paper.

Put the butter, chocolate and crunchy peanut butter into a small saucepan set over low heat and warm until just melted. In a separate saucepan, gently warm through the smooth peanut butter.

Meanwhile, put the eggs, sugar and salt into a large bowl and whisk until combined. Using a rubber spatula, stir in the melted chocolate mixture and flour.

Scrape the mixture into the prepared tin. Drizzle over the smooth peanut butter in 3–4 straight lines, then 'drag' through the peanut butter with the tip of a sharp knife to create a marbled effect.

Bake for 18–20 minutes, until the cake is just firm to the touch, but has a slightly fudgy texture. Leave to cool in the tin for 1–2 minutes, then lift out the block on to a board using the lining paper and cut it into 12–16 squares. Serve warm or cold.

100g (3½oz) unsalted
butter, softened

50g (1¾oz) caster sugar

grated zest of 1 orange

25g (1oz) cocoa powder

50g (2oz) gluten-free
plain flour

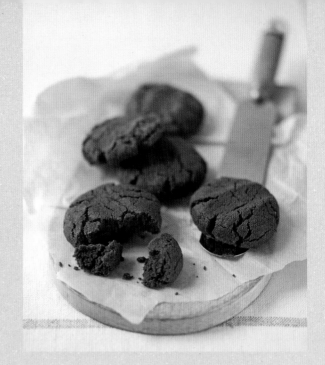

CHOCOLATE ORANGE SHORTBREAD

**PREPARATION TIME: 10 MINUTES,
PLUS CHILLING AND COOLING
COOKING TIME: 15 MINUTES
SERVES: 4**

Preheat the oven to 190°C (375°F), Gas Mark 5. Line a baking sheet with baking paper.

Cream together the butter, sugar and orange zest in a large bowl until the mixture is light and fluffy.

Mix in the cocoa powder and flour and bring the mixture together into a ball of dough. Cover the bowl with clingfilm and chill for 10 minutes.

Shape the mixture into walnut-sized balls and place these on the prepared baking sheet, ensuring they are well spaced. Bake for 5 minutes. Remove the baking sheet from the oven and lightly press down each ball of dough with your finger. Return the baking sheet to the oven and bake for a further 5–7 minutes, until the shortbread has started to become crisp on top.

Transfer to a wire rack and leave to cool completely.

150g (5½oz) plain dark chocolate (85 per cent cocoa solids), broken into pieces

125ml (4fl oz) coconut cream

1 tablespoon mint leaves

125g (4½oz) raspberries

½ teaspoon cocoa powder

½ teaspoon icing sugar

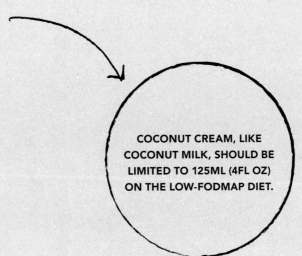

COCONUT CREAM, LIKE COCONUT MILK, SHOULD BE LIMITED TO 125ML (4FL OZ) ON THE LOW-FODMAP DIET.

ULTRA-RICH CHOCOLATE STACKS

PREPARATION TIME: 20 MINUTES, PLUS CHILLING

SERVES: 4

Line a baking sheet with nonstick baking paper.

Put the chocolate pieces into a heatproof bowl and set it over a saucepan of gently simmering water, ensuring the water does not touch the base of the bowl. Stir until melted.

Spoon 12 spoonfuls of the melted chocolate on to the prepared baking sheet and allow each to spread into a disc measuring about 7cm (2¾ inches) in diameter. Refrigerate for 30 minutes until set.

Whip the coconut cream in a bowl until thick. Layer 3 chocolate discs on each of 4 serving plates with the coconut cream, mint leaves and raspberries.

Mix the cocoa and icing sugar together, then dredge the mixture over the chocolate stacks to serve.

175g (6oz) butter, softened, plus extra for greasing

175g (6oz) caster sugar

175g (6oz) brown rice flour, plus extra for dusting

3 eggs

1 tablespoon baking powder

few drops of vanilla extract

1 tablespoon lactose-free or plant-based milk (limit soya to 60ml/4 tablespoons per portion), or standard milk if you know you tolerate lactose

TO DECORATE

4 tablespoons raspberry jam

icing sugar

VICTORIA SANDWICH CAKE

PREPARATION TIME: 10 MINUTES,
**   PLUS COOLING**
COOKING TIME: 20 MINUTES
SERVES: 12

Preheat the oven to 200°C (400°F), Gas Mark 6. Grease and flour 2 x 18cm (7 inch) round cake tins.

Put all the cake ingredients into the bowl of a food processor and whizz until smooth. (Alternatively, beat the ingredients together in a large bowl until the mixture is light and fluffy.)

Spoon the mixture into the prepared tins and bake for about 20 minutes, until risen and golden. Transfer to a wire rack to cool.

Sandwich the cooled cakes together with the jam and dust with icing sugar.

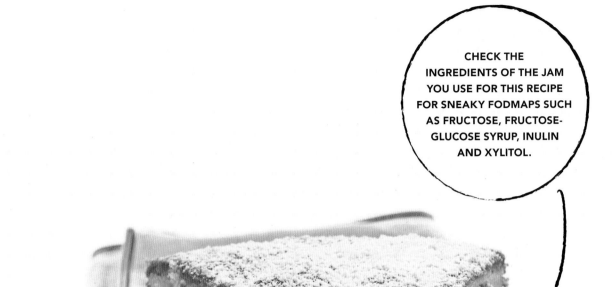

CHECK THE INGREDIENTS OF THE JAM YOU USE FOR THIS RECIPE FOR SNEAKY FODMAPS SUCH AS FRUCTOSE, FRUCTOSE-GLUCOSE SYRUP, INULIN AND XYLITOL.

300g (10½oz) good-quality
dark chocolate with chilli
(70 per cent cocoa solids),
broken into pieces

150g (5½oz) unsalted
butter, diced

6 eggs, separated

125g (4½oz) caster sugar

FOR THE CHILLI SYRUP

1 red chilli, deseeded
and thinly sliced

grated zest and juice
of 1 lime

100g (3½oz) golden
caster sugar

150ml (¼ pint) water

HIGH-FAT FOODS
CAN CAUSE A FLARE
UP IN GASTROINTESTINAL
SYMPTOMS, EVEN IF THEY
ARE LOW IN FODMAPS,
SO STICK TO A MODERATE
SLIVER OF THIS
DELICIOUS DESSERT.

CHOCOLATE & CHILLI MOUSSE CAKE

**PREPARATION TIME: 20 MINUTES,
PLUS COOLING AND CHILLING
COOKING TIME: 35 MINUTES
SERVES: 8–10**

Preheat the oven to 180°C (350°F), Gas Mark 4. Line the base of a 20cm (8 inch) springform cake tin with nonstick baking paper.

Melt the chocolate and butter in a heatproof bowl set over a saucepan of gently simmering water, stirring occasionally, ensuring the water does not touch the base of the bowl.

Meanwhile, whisk the egg yolks with the sugar in a bowl until pale and thick. Stir in the melted chocolate mixture.

Whisk the egg whites in a separate large, grease-free bowl until they form soft peaks. Using a metal spoon, fold a couple of tablespoons of the egg white into the chocolate mixture to loosen it, then fold in the remaining egg white. Pour the mixture into the prepared tin and bake for 20 minutes. Remove the tin from the oven, cover it with kitchen foil (to prevent a crust from forming) and leave to cool. Chill in the refrigerator for at least 4 hours or overnight.

To make the syrup, combine all the ingredients in a small saucepan and heat over low heat, stirring, until the sugar has dissolved. Bring to a boil, then simmer for 10 minutes, until syrupy. Leave to cool.

Remove the cake from the refrigerator 30 minutes before serving in slices, with the syrup poured over.

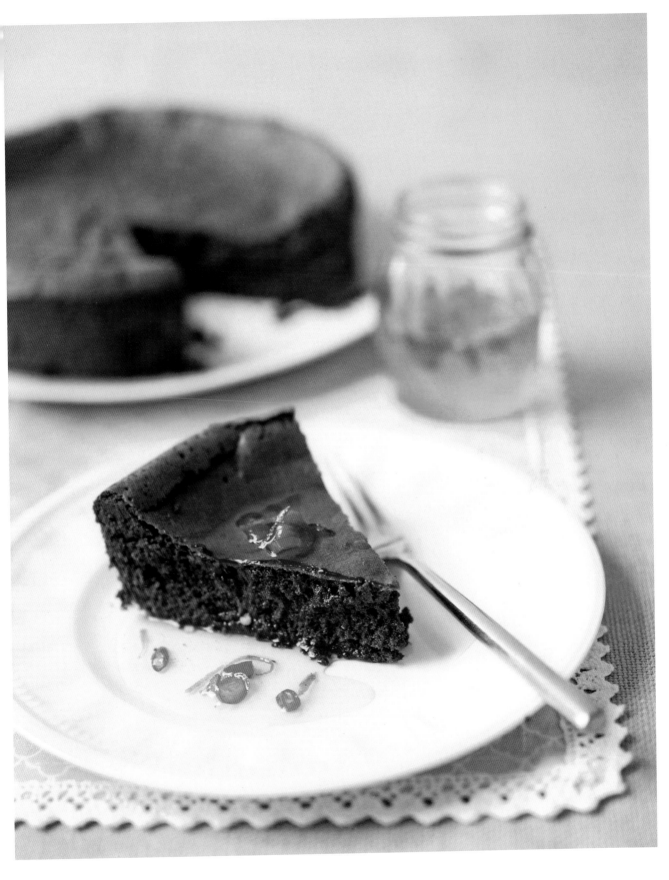

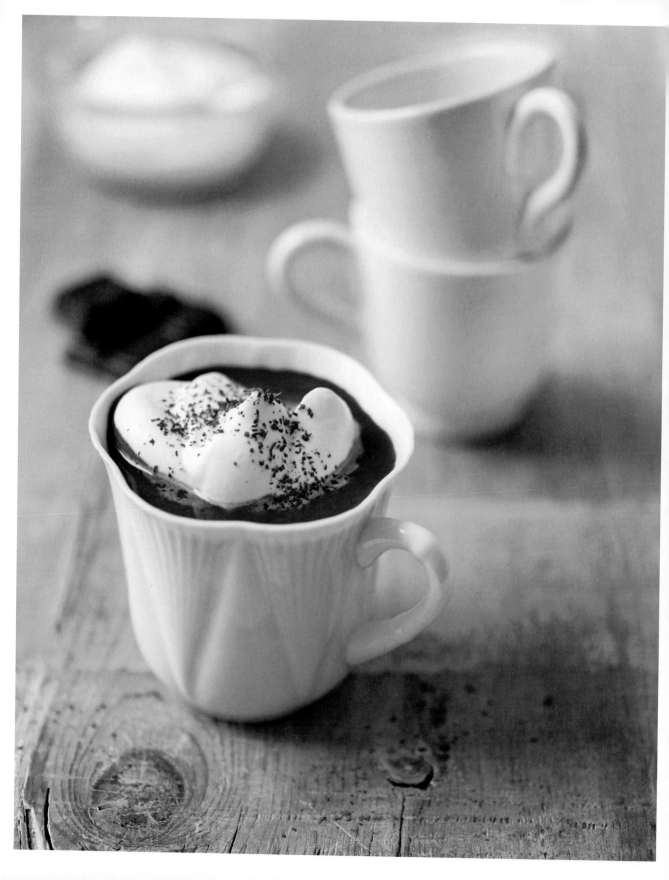

IF USING COCONUT MILK, REDUCE THE QUANTITY TO 125ML (4FL OZ) PER PORTION. LACTOSE-FREE MILKS CAN BE ENJOYED IN UNLIMITED AMOUNTS.

175g (6oz) plain dark chocolate, broken into pieces

1 large pinch of chilli powder

2 tablespoons caster sugar

2 large pinches of ground cinnamon

2 vanilla pods, split lengthways

600ml (20fl oz) milk, or lactose-free or plant-based milk (due to recommended portion limitations you cannot substitute soya milk for this recipe)

200ml (7fl oz) whipping cream, whipped

grated plain dark chocolate, to serve (limit each portion to 45g/1½oz)

CHILLI HOT CHOCOLATE

PREPARATION TIME: 10 MINUTES
COOKING TIME: 5 MINUTES
SERVES: 4

Place the chocolate, chilli powder, sugar, cinnamon, vanilla pods and milk into a pan and heat gently until the chocolate has melted. Bring the mixture to a boil and whisk until the chocolate is very smooth and frothy. Remove the vanilla pods.

Pour the chocolate into 4 warmed mugs and top with the whipped cream and grated chocolate.

INDEX

RESOURCES

USEFUL INFORMATION

King's College London, UK
Information on the low-FODMAP diet from one of the world's leading research and teaching universities:
www.kcl.ac.uk/lsm/research/divisions/dns/projects/fodmaps/faq.aspx

Monash University, Australia
Information on the low-FODMAP diet from the medical researchers who first developed it:
www.med.monash.edu/cecs/gastro/fodmap/

The National Institute of Clinical Excellence (NICE), UK
Provides information for IBS sufferers about their condition and what support they can expect from health professionals in the UK:
www.nice.org.uk/guidance/CG61/ifp/chapter/About-this-information

The IBS Network
UK charity supporting people living with IBS – formally known as The Gut Trust:
www.theibsnetwork.org

FIND A DIETITIAN

When looking for a dietitian, check with the individual practitioner that they are able to advise on the low-FODMAP diet.

For a registered dietitian in the UK who received training from King's College London about the low-FODMAP diet:
www.kcl.ac.uk/lsm/research/divisions/dns/projects/fodmaps/faq.aspx

For a registered dietitian in the UK who works in private practice and specializes in the low-FODMAP diet:
www.freelancedietitians.org (filter the results for dietitians specializing in the low-FODMAP diet).

For a dietitian specializing in the low-FODMAP diet worldwide:
fodmap-diet.com/find-a-fodmap-dietitian/

For a registered dietitian in America:
www.eatright.org/find-an-expert

For a registered dietitian in Canada:
www.dietitians.ca/Your-Health/Find-A-Dietitian/Find-a-Dietitian.aspx

For a registered dietitian in Australia:
daa.asn.au/find-an-apd/

For a registered dietitian in New Zealand:
dietitians.org.nz/find-a-dietitian/

For a registered dietitian in Ireland:
https://www.indi.ie/find-a-dietitian.html

THE REINTRODUCTION PHASE

Re-challenging and Reintroducing FODMAPs: A self-help guide to the entire reintroduction phase of the low FODMAP diet by Lee Martin (CreateSpace Independent Publishing Platform, 2016). A useful guide to the reintroduction phase of the low-FODMAP diet.

APPS

FODMAP by FM (FoodMaestro)
Developed in partnership with medical experts and dietitians from Kings College London and Guy's and St Thomas' NHS Trust, this app helps you to discover FODMAP-friendly foods you can eat, record and track gut symptoms, scan product barcodes to check suitability and create a personalized dietary profile. It also gives portion guidance and includes a FODMAP look-up table.

The Monash University Low FODMAP Diet
Developed for use by researchers at Monash University, Australia, this app assists in the management of the gastrointestinal symptoms associated with IBS. It works on a traffic light system to indicate which foods are suitable for a low-FODMAP diet.

ACKNOWLEDGEMENTS

I would like to thank the team at King's College London for heading up such fantastic work on the research and dissemination of the low-FODMAP diet in the UK. I know you all work so hard to design and undertake clinical trials, train dietitians and develop resources to help health professionals and patients get the most out of the low-FODMAP diet. It was the team at King's College London who put FODMAPs on my radar back in the late 2000s and I have since learned so much from their expertise and their published research.

I would also like to thank Imperial College NHS Trust for supporting me from the very beginning in setting up a low-FODMAP service and run a dedicated clinic to help those with functional bowel disorders.

Thank you to Octopus Publishing who have worked so hard on this book and got it to print in such a short time frame.

Last but definitely not least I would like to thank my patients whom I admire so much for working so hard to improve their symptoms: seeing you improve brings me so much joy – I am constantly learning from you.

PICTURE CREDITS